Obesity, Diabetes, and Adrenal Disorders

Guest Editor

THOMAS K. GRAVES, DVM, PhD

VETERINARY CLINICS OF NORTH AMERICA: SMALL ANIMAL PRACTICE

www.vetsmall.theclinics.com

March 2010 • Volume 40 • Number 2

SAUNDERS an imprint of ELSEVIER, Inc.

W.B. SAUNDERS COMPANY
A Division of Elsevier Inc.

1600 John F. Kennedy Blvd. ● Suite 1800 ● Philadelphia, PA 19103-2899
http://www.vetsmall.theclinics.com

VETERINARY CLINICS OF NORTH AMERICA: SMALL ANIMAL PRACTICE Volume 40, Number 2
March 2010 ISSN 0195-5616, ISBN-13: 978-1-4377-1887-4

Editor: John Vassallo; j.vassallo@elsevier.com
Developmental Editor: Theresa Collier

Veterinary Clinics of North America: Small Animal Practice (ISSN 0195-5616) is published bimonthly (For Post Office use only: volume 40 issue 2 of 6) by Elsevier Inc., 360 Park Avenue South, New York, NY 10010-1710. Months of issue are January, March, May, July, September, and November. Business and Editorial Offices: 1600 John F. Kennedy Blvd., Ste. 1800, Philadelphia, PA 19103-2899. Customer Service Office: 3251 Riverport Lane, Maryland Heights, MO 63043. Periodicals postage paid at New York, NY and additional mailing offices. Subscription prices are $245.00 per year (domestic individuals), $388.00 per year (domestic institutions), $122.00 per year (domestic students/residents), $324.00 per year (Canadian individuals), $477.00 per year (Canadian institutions), $360.00 per year (international individuals), $477.00 per year (international institutions), and $177.00 per year (international and Canadian students/residents). To receive student/resident rate, orders must be accompanied by name of affiliated institution, date of term, and the *signature* of program/residency coordinator on institution letterhead. Orders will be billed at individual rate until proof of status is received. Foreign air speed delivery is included in all *Clinics* subscription prices. All prices are subject to change without notice. **POSTMASTER:** Send address changes to *Veterinary Clinics of North America: Small Animal Practice*, Elsevier Health Sciences Division, Subscription Customer Service, 3251 Riverport Lane, Maryland Heights, MO 63043. Customer Service (orders, claims, online, change of address): Elsevier Periodicals Customer Service, Elsevier Health Sciences Division Subscription Customer Service 3251 Riverport Lane Maryland Heights, MO 63043. Tel: 1-800-654-2452 (U.S. and Canada); 314-447-8871 (outside U.S. and Canada). Fax: 314-447-8029. E-mail: journalscustomerservice-usa@elsevier.com (for print support); journalsonlinesupport-usa@elsevier.com (for online support).

Reprints. For copies of 100 or more of articles in this publication, please contact the Commercial Reprints Department, Elsevier Inc., 360 Park Avenue South, New York, NY 10010-1710. Tel.: 212-633-3812; Fax: 212-462-1935; E-mail: reprints@elsevier.com.

Veterinary Clinics of North America: Small Animal Practice is also published in Japanese by Inter Zoo Publishing Co., Ltd., Aoyama Crystal-Bldg 5F, 3-5-12 Kitaaoyama, Minato-ku, Tokyo 107-0061, Japan.

Veterinary Clinics of North America: Small Animal Practice is covered in *Current Contents/Agriculture, Biology and Environmental Sciences, Science Citation Index, ASCA, MEDLINE/PubMed (Index Medicus), Excerpta Medica,* and *BIOSIS.*

Printed and bound by CPI Group (UK) Ltd, Croydon, CR0 4YY

Transferred to Digital Print 2011

Contributors

GUEST EDITOR

THOMAS K. GRAVES, DVM, PhD
Diplomate, American College of Veterinary Internal Medicine; Associate Professor
of Small Animal Medicine; Assistant Department Head for Curriculum and Instruction,
Department of Veterinary Clinical Medicine, University of Illinois College of Veterinary
Medicine, Urbana, Illinois

AUTHORS

ELLEN N. BEHREND, VMD, PhD
Diplomate, American College of Veterinary Internal Medicine; Professor, Department
of Clinical Sciences, College of Veterinary Medicine, Auburn University, Auburn, Alabama

SARA GALAC, DVM
Assistant Professor, Department of Clinical Sciences of Companion Animals, Faculty
of Veterinary Medicine, Utrecht University, Utrecht, The Netherlands

CHEN GILOR, DVM
Diplomate, American College of Veterinary Internal Medicine; Research Fellow,
Department of Veterinary Clinical Medicine, University of Illinois College of Veterinary
Medicine, Urbana, Illinois

THOMAS K. GRAVES, DVM, PhD
Diplomate, American College of Veterinary Internal Medicine; Associate Professor of
Small Animal Medicine; Assistant Department Head for Curriculum and Instruction,
Department of Veterinary Clinical Medicine, University of Illinois College of Veterinary
Medicine, Urbana, Illinois

REBECKA S. HESS, DVM
Diplomate, American College of Veterinary Internal Medicine; Associate Professor
of Internal Medicine, Department of Clinical Studies-Philadelphia, School of Veterinary
Medicine, University of Pennsylvania, Philadelphia, Pennsylvania

ROBERT KENNIS, DVM, MS
Diplomate, American College of Veterinary Dermatology; Associate Professor,
Department of Clinical Sciences, College of Veterinary Medicine, Auburn University,
Auburn, Alabama

DONG YONG KIL, PhD
Department of Animal Sciences, University of Illinois, Urbana, Illinois

HANS S. KOOISTRA, DVM, PhD
Diplomate, European College of Veterinary Internal Medicine-Companion Animals;
Associate Professor, Department of Clinical Sciences of Companion Animals, Faculty
of Veterinary Medicine, Utrecht University, Utrecht, The Netherlands

MAURIA A. O'BRIEN, DVM
Diplomate, American College of Veterinary Emergency and Critical Care; Clinical Assistant Professor, Department of Veterinary Clinical Medicine, University of Illinois College of Veterinary Medicine, Urbana, Illinois

IAN K. RAMSEY, BVSc, PhD
Diplomate, European College of Veterinary Internal Medicine (Companion Animals); RCVS Specialist and Diplomate in Small Animal Medicine, Professor of Small Animal Medicine, Faculty of Veterinary Medicine, University of Glasgow, Bearsden, Glasgow, United Kingdom

CLAUDIA E. REUSCH, DVM
Diplomate, European College of Veterinary Internal Medicine (Companion Animals) Clinic for Small Animal Internal Medicine, Vetsuisse Faculty, University of Zurich, Zurich, Switzerland

STEFAN SCHELLENBERG, DVM
Clinic for Small Animal Internal Medicine, Vetsuisse Faculty, University of Zurich, Zurich, Switzerland

RHONDA L. SCHULMAN, DVM
Diplomate, American College of Veterinary Internal Medicine; Animal Specialty Group, Los Angeles, California

J. CATHARINE SCOTT-MONCRIEFF, MS, MA, Vet MB
Diplomate, American College of Veterinary Internal Medicine; Diplomate, European College of Veterinary Internal Medicine; Diplomate, Small Animal Medicine; Professor Internal Medicine and Assistant Department Head, Department of Veterinary Clinical Sciences, VCS/LYNN, Purdue University, West Lafayette, Indiana

KELLY S. SWANSON, PhD
Associate Professor, Department of Animal Sciences, Division of Nutritional Sciences, University of Illinois; Adjunct Assistant Professor, Department of Veterinary Clinical Medicine, University of Illinois College of Veterinary Medicine, Urbana, Illinois

MONIQUE WENGER, DVM
Diplomate, American College of Veterinary Internal Medicine; Diplomate, European College of Veterinary Internal Medicine-Companion Animals; Clinic for Small Animal Internal Medicine, Vetsuisse Faculty, University of Zurich, Zurich, Switzerland

DEBRA L. ZORAN, DVM, PhD
Diplomate, American College of Veterinary Internal Medicine (Small Animal Internal Medicine); Associate Professor and Chief of Medicine, Department of Small Animal Clinical Sciences, College of Veterinary Medicine and Biomedical Sciences, Texas A&M University, College Station, Texas

Contents

There are several recent advances in the diagnosis of Cushing's syndrome, or spontaneous hypercortisolism, in dogs. Diagnostic procedures are being reshaped by the recognition of new causes of the disease and advances in imaging procedures. This article reviews the clinical manifestations, diagnostic procedures, and the forms and causes of the syndrome.

Over the last 10 years, trilostane, a competitive inhibitor of steroid synthesis, is being widely used for the treatment of canine hyperadrenocorticism. Trilostane causes a significant but reversible decrease in cortisol production and a concomitant improvement in clinical signs in most dogs with this common condition. Side effects, though infrequent, can be serious: dogs treated with this drug require regular monitoring. This review summarizes current knowledge of the use of this drug with particular emphasis on its efficacy, safety, adverse reactions, and effects on endocrine parameters. Brief mention is made of its other uses in dogs and other species.

In the past 5 to 10 years, much interest has arisen in the syndrome of occult hyperadrenocorticism. Patients with occult hyperadrenocorticism purportedly have many clinical signs and routine laboratory abnormalities suggestive of the presence of typical hyperadrenocorticism, or Cushing's syndrome (ie, hypercortisolism either due to a pituitary or adrenal tumor). However, the standard diagnostic tests—corticotropin (ACTH) stimulation and low-dose dexamethasone suppression tests—are normal. A theory has arisen that the clinical signs of occult hyperadrenocorticism are due to excess adrenal secretion of sex hormones rather than cortisol. The authors believe that the role of sex hormones has not been proven. The article reviews the evidence both for and against the importance of sex hormones in creating occult hyperadrenocorticism.

Human recombinant synthetic insulin analogs allow better control of blood glucose concentrations while minimizing the risk of hypoglycemic events in diabetic human patients. Little information is available regarding the use of insulin analogs in cats and dogs. Insulin lispro is an ultrashort-acting analog that has been used in the intensive treatment of dogs with diabetic ketoacidosis. Insulin glargine and insulin detemir are long-acting, and are used in people as basal insulin replacement. Both are associated with reduced risk of hypoglycemia, while detemir also is associated with less undesired weight gain. In cats, insulin detemir and insulin glargine have longer durations of action than traditionally used insulin formulations, and both have been used successfully in once-a-day regimens for treatment of diabetes. Insulins detemir and glargine may have shorter durations of action in cats than in people, and more variability in their effects.

In diabetic dogs, many concurrent diseases can cause resistance to exogenous insulin. The most common concurrent disorders in diabetic dogs are hyperadrenocorticism, urinary tract infection, acute pancreatitis, neoplasia, and hypothyroidism. When a concurrent disorder is treated, the insulin dose should be decreased to avoid possible hypoglycemia when an underlying cause of insulin resistance is removed. Hormonal disturbances have been observed in obese dogs, but the clinical significance of these changes is not known.

Diabetic ketoacidosis and hyperglycemic hyperosmolar syndrome are two serious and potentially life-threatening complications of diabetes mellitus. Understanding pathophysiology is crucial to the proper management of veterinary patients with these disorders. This article reviews the biochemical alterations contributing to these conditions, and discusses traditional and controversial management strategies.

Hypertension is classified as idiopathic or secondary. In animals with idiopathic hypertension, persistently elevated blood pressure is not caused by an identifiable underlying or predisposing disease. Until recently, more than 95% of cases of hypertension in humans were diagnosed as idiopathic. New studies have shown, however, a much higher prevalence of secondary causes, such as primary hyperaldosteronism. In dogs and cats, secondary hypertension is the most prevalent form and is subclassified into renal and endocrine hypertension. This review focuses on the most common causes of endocrine hypertension in dogs and cats.

Primary hyperaldosteronism (PHA) is being recognized more frequently in cats. Usual hallmarks of the disease include hypokalemia and systemic hypertension. Ultrasound frequently detects an abnormality in the affected adrenal gland. Diagnosis is based on increased plasma or serum aldosterone concentrations, particularly in the face of hypokalemia and low renin

activity (when measurement is available). Cats with PHA have good prognoses with surgical excision of tumor-bearing adrenal glands. Medical
management can stabilize patients for many months. The reported incidence is likely to increase as practitioners become more aware of the condition and diagnose it earlier in the disease course. If veterinarians choose
to use humans as an experimental model, PHA should be considered a differential for cats with hypertension of unknown cause or that is refractory
to treatment. Using hypokalemia as a definitive criterion in screening for
PHA may result in late-stage diagnosis and underrecognition of incidence
of PHA in the hypertensive population.

FORTHCOMING ISSUES

May 2010
Immunology and Vaccinology
Melissa A. Kennedy, DVM, PhD,
Guest Editor

July 2010
Topics in Cardiology
Jonathan A. Abbott, DVM,
Guest Editor

September 2010
Spinal Disorders
Ronaldo C. da Costa, DMV, MSc, PhD,
Guest Editor

RECENT ISSUES

January 2010
Diseases of the Brain
William B. Thomas, DVM, MS,
Guest Editor

November 2009
Small Animal Parasites: Biology and Control
David S. Lindsay, PhD and
Anne M. Zajac, DVM, PhD,
Guest Editors

September 2009
Endoscopy
Mary-Ann G. Radlinsky, DVM, MS,
Guest Editor

RELATED INTEREST
Veterinary Clinics of North America: Exotic Animal Practice
January 2008 (Vol. 11, No. 1)
Endocrinology
Anthony A. Pilny, DVM, Dipl., ABVP—Avian, *Guest Editor*

THE CLINICS ARE NOW AVAILABLE ONLINE!

Access your subscription at:
www.theclinics.com

Preface

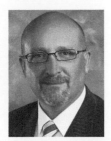

Thomas K. Graves, DVM, PhD
Guest Editor

Obesity, diabetes, and adrenal disease occupy major, overlapping tracts on the constantly changing landscape of small animal medicine. The incidence of diabetes in dogs and cats has increased steadily over the past few decades, and the veterinary clinician is constantly challenged by developments in human diabetes therapy that affect our ability to treat our patients. The human obesity epidemic has reached historic proportions and is mirrored by obesity in the pet population. As with diabetes and obesity, there are important recent developments, some controversial, in canine hypercortisolism, a disorder closely associated with both diabetes and obesity.

Many important problems are addressed in this issue. Herein is new information on the endocrinology of adipose tissue, and this provides clear evidence to support the view of obesity as a disease. Current and comprehensive overviews of diagnosis and treatment of canine Cushing's syndrome are expertly presented, and the controversy of "atypical Cushing's syndrome" is discussed in an evidence-based and balanced manner. The issue explores the intersection of diabetes and adrenal disease, and the complexities of endocrine hypertension, aldosterone, and diabetic ketoacidosis. Human insulin analogs, dominant players in human diabetes therapy and increasingly important in veterinary medicine, are reviewed here as well.

Working with this list of expert authors has been a powerful learning experience for me, and I am grateful to each and every one of them for their hard work and knowledge. I am confident that readers will find new information and new points of view in these pages, and I hope concepts presented here will spark new clinical research ideas and will advance the way we care for dogs and cats with complex endocrine conditions.

Thomas K. Graves, DVM, PhD
Department of Veterinary Clinical Medicine
University of Illinois College of Veterinary Medicine
1008 West Hazelwood Drive
Urbana, IL 61802, USA

E-mail address:
tgraves@illinois.edu

Vet Clin Small Anim 40 (2010) xi
doi:10.1016/j.cvsm.2009.12.002
0195-5616/10/$ – see front matter © 2010 Elsevier Inc. All rights reserved.

Endocrinology of Obesity

Dong Yong Kil, PhD[a], Kelly S. Swanson, PhD[b,c],*

KEYWORDS

- Obesity • Dogs • Cats • Endocrinology
- Hormonal abnormalities

Obesity is defined as a clinical state of excessive accumulation of body fat. Currently, obesity is considered one of the most important human health concerns, both in the industrialized and developing countries, because it is highly associated with type 2 diabetes mellitus, hypertension, hyperlipidemia, and heart diseases.[1] Although obesity and associated metabolic disorders have been primarily implicated in human health, they are now a growing concern in dogs and cats. In the United States, approximately 35% of adult dogs and cats are overweight or obese.[2,3] As observed in humans, canine and feline obesity are mainly caused by positive energy balance. Obese dogs and cats have a decreased life span and multiple metabolic disorders.[4]

Obesity serves as a direct or indirect cause of various endocrine abnormalities contributing to metabolic disorders. The development of obesity may also be secondary to endocrine disorders in dogs and cats.[5] However, the cause-effect relationship between obesity and endocrine alterations is often unclear. This review focuses on the role of endocrine organs and alterations in response to obesity in humans, dogs, and cats. Although a lack of information on obesity-induced endocrine alterations in dogs and cats exists in the literature, we have attempted to include all relevant published data in these species.

HYPOTHALAMUS AND PITUITARY GLANDS

The hypothalamic-pituitary axis is a neuroendocrine system that regulates various body functions, such as stress responsiveness, the immune response, and energy

[a] Department of Animal Sciences, University of Illinois, 180 Animal Sciences Laboratory, 1207 West Gregory Drive, Urbana, IL 61801, USA
[b] Department of Animal Sciences, Division of Nutritional Sciences, University of Illinois, 162 Animal Sciences Laboratory, 1207 West Gregory Drive, Urbana, IL 61801, USA
[c] Department of Veterinary Clinical Medicine, University of Illinois, 162 Animal Sciences Laboratory, 1207 West Gregory Drive, Urbana, IL 61801, USA
* Corresponding author. Department of Animal Sciences, Division of Nutritional Sciences, University of Illinois, 162 Animal Sciences Laboratory, 1207 West Gregory Drive, Urbana, IL 61001.
E-mail address: ksswanso@illinois.edu (K.S. Swanson).

Vet Clin Small Anim 40 (2010) 205–219
doi:10.1016/j.cvsm.2009.10.004
0195-5616/10/$ – see front matter © 2010 Elsevier Inc. All rights reserved.

homeostasis. Under control of the hypothalamus, the anterior pituitary produces several hormones that act on target cells of other endocrine organs.

Growth hormone (GH) is secreted from the anterior pituitary, and its secretion is regulated by the hypothalamic hormones growth hormone–releasing hormone (GHRH) and somatostatin. The main function of GH is to enhance growth in young animals. GH plays a role in increasing muscle mass, decreasing body fat, and increasing bone mineralization in adult humans and animals. Numerous studies in humans and rodents indicate that obesity results in a marked decrease in plasma GH concentrations, representing GH deficiency.[6–8] It appears that impaired GH secretion is a consequence of obesity because weight loss restores the defect in GH secretion.[9,10] It is speculated that this GH deficiency results from diminished pituitary somatotroph responsiveness to GH stimuli, hyposecretion of GHRH, and hypersecretion of somatostatin.[10] Hyperinsulinemia and increased plasma free fatty acids associated with obesity also contribute to GH deficiency.[8,11] Obesity elevates circulating growth hormone–binding protein (GHBP) concentrations, which may be an adaptive mechanism to increase GH sensitivity in obese subjects.[12]

Insulin-like growth factor I (IGF-I) is produced by various tissues, mainly the liver, and acts as a physiologic mediator of GH action. Plasma IGF-I concentrations are variable in obese humans but may be expected to be decreased because of GH deficiency.[10,13] However, obesity-induced hyperinsulinemia may decrease the expression of IGF-binding protein, thereby increasing free IGF-I concentrations that may exacerbate GH deficiency via the feedback inhibition.[7,14] In dogs, obesity induced by prolonged overfeeding resulted in increased plasma IGF-I concentrations, which was positively correlated with hyperinsulinemia.[15] In another study of naturally acquired obesity, serum IGF-I concentrations were 80% greater in obese dogs as compared with lean dogs.[16] In another study, however, only 20% of obese dogs had elevated serum IGF-I concentrations, demonstrating little correlation with body weight.[17]

Corticotropin-releasing hormone (CRH) produced by the hypothalamus stimulates the adrenal gland to secrete cortisol via the activation of corticotropin (ACTH) release from the pituitary gland. Obesity is suggested to be the cause of a hyperactive hypothalamic-pituitary-adrenal (HPA) axis. In obese rodents, both plasma corticosterone concentrations and the response of corticosterone and ACTH to exogenous stressors were greatly elevated as compared with lean controls.[18] Hyperactivity of the HPA axis was also observed in obese humans.[13,19] However, the stimulatory effect of ACTH on cortisol secretion was decreased with obesity; the increase in ACTH was relatively greater than that of cortisol secretion.[20] Hyperactivity of the HPA axis may be affected by the location of fat deposition because central obesity induces greater activity of the HPA axis than does peripheral obesity.[21] Increased leptin concentrations in obese individuals may also contribute to a hyperactive HPA axis because of leptin's stimulatory effect on CRH and ACTH production.[20] The effect of obesity on the activity of the HPA axis in dogs is not clear. One study reported that only 4 of 31 obese dogs had a hypersecretion of cortisol after intramuscular ACTH injection.[17]

Thyrotropin-releasing hormone (TRH), secreted from the hypothalamus, stimulates the anterior pituitary gland to release thyrotropin (TSH), which subsequently activates secretion of thyroxine (T_4) and triiodothyronine (T_3) from the thyroid gland. The hypothalamic-pituitary-thyroid gland (HPT) axis plays an important role in energy homeostasis by modulating basal metabolic rate. Thus, thyroid hormone deficiency decreases basal energy expenditure, which may be a direct cause of obesity.[13,22] Hypothyroidism is also a risk factor for canine obesity.[5] In humans, however, obesity induces little change in the basal activity of the HPT axis, although the results are variable.[13,23,24] Like humans, obese dogs generally have normal thyroid function despite having slightly increased plasma concentrations of total T_4 and T_3.[16,25] On the contrary, one study reported that obesity caused increased TSH and decreased free T_4 concentrations in dogs, changes that often indicate subclinical hypothyroidism.[17] Elevated free serum T_4 concentrations, but normal total T_4 and TSH concentrations have been reported in obese cats.[26] Thyroid hormone resistance may contribute to altered activity of the HPT axis observed in obese humans and animals.[26–28] Increased leptin concentrations may also be responsible for modulating the activity of the HPT axis because it is thought to stimulate TRH and, consequently, thyroid hormone production.[27,29] The cause-effect relationship between obesity and thyroid dysfunction, however, still remains a question in humans and animals.

Prolactin is secreted from the anterior pituitary, with its secretion being controlled by prolactin-releasing hormone (PRH), dopamine, and TRH from the hypothalamus. Prolactin not only has functions pertaining to reproduction and lactation, but also in immune response, osmoregulation, and angiogenesis. In general, basal prolactin secretion is normal in obese humans.[24] However, one study of obese women reported that serum prolactin concentrations were elevated with increased body mass index and that prolactin secretion rates were specifically associated with visceral fat mass.[30] Decreased dopaminergic tone, which normally inhibits prolactin secretion, and increased leptin concentrations via its stimulator effects may contribute to increased prolactin concentrations in obese subjects.[30,31] Moreover, obesity may blunt prolactin responsiveness to various stimuli.[32] It was reported that obese women had decreased responsiveness to TRH stimulation, demonstrated by decreased prolactin production rates to TRH administration as compared with normal-weight women.[33] Similar results have been observed in children with mild to moderate obesity.[34] Increased prolactin concentrations have also been reported in obese dogs and cats.[17,35]

Obesity influences reproductive functions in both men and women by altering the activity of the hypothalamic-pituitary-gonadal axis.[36] Adipose tissue also acts as a reservoir of sex hormones. Therefore, obesity may modulate circulating concentrations of sex hormones and the relative ratio of estrogens and androgens.[37] In obese men, total and free testosterone concentrations decrease as body weight increases.[36,38] Reduced testosterone concentrations with obesity may be attributed to decreased sex hormone–binding globulin (SHBG) and gonadotropin concentrations.[36,38] On the contrary, obese women are often reported to show hyperandrogenism as evidenced by increased testosterone and decreased SHBG concentrations.[39] Similar alterations in circulating testosterone concentrations have been observed in obese male and female dogs.[16] This dichotomy is difficult to explain, but is partly a result of different HPA axis activity between the sexes.[19]

Estrogen concentrations tend to be increased in both obese male and female humans probably because expanding adipose tissue elevates the conversion of androgen precursors into estrogen.[40] Data pertaining to obesity-induced alterations of sex hormones in dogs and cats are scarce. Moreover, the frequent practice of neutering dogs and cats, which is a risk factor for obesity, further complicates the relationship between obesity and sex hormones because it leads to a distinguished state of hormonal homeostasis. For instance, neutering dogs increases luteinizing hormone concentrations because of the absence of negative feedback from androgens and estrogens as well as an alteration of the pituitary response to gonadotropin-releasing hormones.[41,42] Similar results are expected in neutered cats.[35]

PANCREATIC HORMONES

Insulin is produced by β cells in the islet of Langerhans of the pancreas and is characterized as an anabolic hormone. Insulin resistance and hyperinsulinemia are well known characteristics of human obesity.[40] Similarly, obesity contributes to insulin dysfunction in dogs and cats although the relationship between obesity and insulin function differs between the 2 species.[43] In cats, it has been reported that obesity decreases insulin sensitivity by approximately 50%.[44] Weight reduction corrects impaired insulin sensitivity and hyperinsulinemia in overweight cats.[45,46] It has been calculated that each kilogram of weight gain reduces insulin sensitivity and glucose effectiveness in cats by 30%.[46] Obese male cats may be more prone to diabetes than obese females because of a lower innate insulin sensitivity and higher basal insulin concentrations.[44] Obese dogs also develop insulin resistance and hyperinsulinemia and are responsive to weight loss, which leads to a recovery of insulin sensitivity and decreased insulin concentrations.[15,16,47] Obesity is also associated with pancreatitis in dogs, although no cause and effect has been established, and therefore may lead to an increased risk for developing type I diabetes.[48]

High fat-induced obesity in dogs decreases insulin accessibility to skeletal muscle, resulting in decreased insulin sensitivity.[49] Visceral obesity results in greater insulin resistance and hyperinsulinemia than peripheral obesity in human beings,[47] but it is not known if the same holds true for dogs and cats. Increased concentrations of free fatty acids and inflammatory cytokines, such as tumor necrosis factor-α (TNF-α) and interleukin-6 (IL-6), produced by visceral fat are thought to be possible reasons for this observation.[15,47] Increased leptin concentrations may also contribute to insulin resistance by impairing insulin function in various insulin-dependent tissues.[50] Insulin resistance with diet-induced obesity also appears to be more pronounced in adult or mature dogs than in young dogs.[51]

Glucagon is produced by pancreatic α cells and is known as an antagonistic hormone of insulin. Therefore, hyperinsulinemia secondary to obesity may be expected to decrease glucagon production. However, there is evidence that glucagon resistance exists in humans and rodents, resulting in increased circulating glucagon concentrations.[52–54] It appears that glucagon resistance derived from obesity is caused by insulin resistance of pancreatic α cells.[55]

Amylin is also produced by pancreatic β cells and is secreted with insulin. Amylin functions with insulin synergistically but has inhibitory effects on glucagon secretion. Thus, amylin secretion following a meal results in a metabolic switch from endogenous glucose production to dietary glucose use.[55] It is reported that plasma amylin concentrations increase in obese humans and decrease after weight loss.[56,57] Increased insulin secretion as a result of insulin resistance may be a cause of increased amylin production.[57] Overexpression of amylin results in pancreatic islet amyloidosis and impairs β-cell function, which may in turn exacerbate insulin dysfunction.[55,57] Given the species similarities as it pertains to insulin resistance, obesity is also expected to elevate amylin concentrations in obese dogs and cats.[58,59]

Pancreatic polypeptide (PP) is secreted primarily by PP cells in the pancreatic islets of Langerhans and functions by suppressing gastric emptying, pancreatic enzyme secretion, and appetite.[60] Decreased PP concentrations have been observed in human obesity, but are normalized after weight loss, indicating that obesity is a causal factor in its reduction.[61–63] In humans, PP concentrations were greater in obese subjects with glucose intolerance as compared with obese subjects with normal glucose tolerance, indicating that insulin sensitivity may be a confounding factor between obesity and plasma PP concentrations.[64] It was also reported that PP secretion, either in response to hypoglycemia or after a meal, was impaired in obese humans.[62,65] However, the underlying mechanisms for low PP concentrations as a consequence of obesity have not been fully elucidated.

ADIPOSE TISSUE

Adipose tissue is composed of numerous cell types, including adipocytes, fibroblasts, macrophages, and endothelial cells. The primary role of adipose tissue is to store energy in the form of lipids. However, adipose tissue is also now appreciated as an active endocrine organ that synthesizes and releases metabolically active substances, termed adipokines, which act systemically or locally to influence various metabolic reactions.[1] Several adipokines such as leptin, adiponectin, and resistin have been identified in humans and animals. Increased fat mass has been implicated in the dysregulation of adipokine production and contributes to various obesity-related metabolic abnormalities.[1,66]

Leptin has been the most widely studied among adipokines in humans and animals. Leptin is known as an antiobesity hormone.[67] In general, leptin functions to decrease food intake, increase energy expenditure, and modulate glucose and fat metabolism through central and peripheral systems.[50] As observed in humans and rodents, plasma leptin concentrations in dogs and cats increase with increasing body fat mass and adipocyte size, and subsequent weight loss leads to decreased leptin concentrations.[16,46,68,69] Therefore, plasma leptin concentration is considered a biomarker for the degree of obesity in dogs and cats, regardless of breed, sex, and age.[70–73] In an early experiment, exogenous leptin administration was shown to reverse obesity in leptin-deficient mice.[74] However, consequent experiments in humans and animals have consistently reported elevated leptin concentrations in obese subjects, emphasizing the leptin resistance that occurs with obesity.[67–69,75]

Leptin is usually thought of as a long-term regulator of body weight. However, it was reported that postprandial plasma leptin concentrations tend to decrease in lean but not obese people, indicating decreased leptin action in the short term as well.[76] Defective leptin receptors or impaired signaling in target tissues may be a cause of decreased leptin sensitivity and leptin resistance.[50] In a canine study, increased serum leptin concentrations but defective leptin transport through the blood-brain barrier was observed as dogs became obese.[73] Plasma leptin is present in a free or a protein-bound form.[77] It has been suggested that an imbalance between free and bound forms of leptin may be associated with increased leptin resistance because free leptin concentrations increase in obese people, whereas most leptin is bound to protein in lean people.[50,77]

Adiponectin is also produced and secreted exclusively from adipose tissue in humans, dogs, and cats.[78–80] Adiponectin has been considered a beneficial adipokine because it improves insulin sensitivity by enhancing fat and carbohydrate oxidation in peripheral tissues, suppressing hepatic gluconeogenesis, and inhibiting inflammatory responses.[66,81,82] Although it is the most abundant adipokine produced by adipose tissue, obesity results in decreased adiponectin gene expression and plasma adiponectin concentrations in humans and rodents.[78,81] Decreased plasma adiponectin concentrations have been observed in dogs with experimentally induced and clinical obesity.[79,83] Likewise, obese cats have significantly lower plasma adiponectin concentrations than normal cats.[46,80] Therefore, it appears that plasma adiponectin, in addition to leptin, can be a biomarker for body condition status in dogs and cats.[79]

It is suggested that defective adiponectin secretion in obesity is caused by increased feedback inhibition from inflammatory cytokines such as TNF-α and IL-6, which are escalated with body fat mass.[84] Moreover, obesity is likely to decrease the expression of adiponectin receptors in both muscle and liver, leading to adiponectin resistance that is highly related to insulin resistance.[85] Alteration in the circulating forms of adiponectin (low molecular weight [LMW] versus high molecular weight [HMW]) may occur during the development of obesity. In morbidly obese humans, the relative ratio of HMW to total adiponectin decreased with obesity but increased after gastric-bypass surgery.[86] Normal levels of HMW adiponectin but decreased levels of LMW adiponectin was also reported in obese humans.[87] The differing molecular weight forms of adiponectin have not been examined in dogs or cats.

Resistin is another adipokine and is induced by adipogenesis, although circulating mononuclear cells (eg, macrophages) are probably the main source of resistin in humans.[88,89] Resistin has gained great attention because of its antagonistic effect on insulin function in mice.[90] Moreover, there is evidence that the level of plasma resistin increases in obese mice and humans.[90,91] In a study with morbidly obese humans, resistin mRNA expression in adipose tissue was increased in obese subjects but was undetectable in lean subjects.[89] However, the relationship between obesity and resistin is still inconclusive in humans. Resistin expression has not been studied in dogs and cats.[66]

Adipose tissues also produce a variety of proinflammatory cytokines such as TNF-α and IL-6, which were originally studied for their role in various immune cells. The primary role of TNF-α and IL-6 is to activate the immune system in response to infection or cancer. However, overproduction of these cytokines has been considered a risk factor in various human diseases. Increased infiltration and accumulation of macrophages in adipose has been observed in obese subjects, which explains the increased expression of TNF-α and IL-6 during the expansion of adipose tissues.[92] Regardless of what cell type is secreting these substances, adipose is appreciated as an active immunologic tissue.[93] It is well known that obesity increases the production and circulating concentrations of both TNF-α and IL-6 and that weight reduction neutralizes them. Therefore, obesity represents a chronic low-grade inflammatory condition.[82,94]

In dogs, markedly increased plasma TNF-α concentrations were observed after 30 weeks of overfeeding as compared with a healthy weight at baseline.[15] The authors observed a 27-fold increase in plasma TNF-α during very rapid weight gain in the first 20 weeks of overfeeding. From weeks 20 to 30, a time at which an obese condition was maintained, plasma TNF-α concentrations tended to decrease but were still 10 times greater than baseline. The reason for decreased plasma TNF-α during the maintenance of obesity is still unclear, but may be attributed to increased activity of peroxisome proliferator activated receptor γ (PPARγ) that has inhibitory effects on TNF-α expression.[15] As observed in dogs, TNF-α expression in adipose tissue and skeletal muscle was much greater in obese than in lean cats.[95,96] Published data in humans and animals consistently indicate that overexpression of TNF-α and IL-6 complicates obesity-associated metabolic syndromes, such as insulin resistance, cardiovascular diseases, and osteoarthritis, via impaired insulin signaling, dyslipidemia, and stimulation of hepatic C-reactive protein.[93,94,97,98]

GASTROINTESTINAL HORMONES

Several hormones are synthesized and released by the gastrointestinal tract (GIT). Although the research focus of these hormones has often been limited to the GIT itself, GIT hormones are now appreciated as active regulators of appetite, satiety, and body energy balance. Therefore, GIT hormones are assumed to be closely linked with the development of obesity and have been implicated in its prevention.

Ghrelin is synthesized primarily by the X/A-like cells in the oxyntic glands of the gastric fundus and is known to stimulate GH release.[99] Plasma ghrelin is present in the circulation in 2 major forms, depending on the acylation of its serine residue by n-octanoic acid.[99] Although deacylated ghrelin is predominant in circulation, acylated ghrelin is known as an active form.[99] Ghrelin has been recognized as the only orexigenic GIT hormone, with concentrations peaking before a meal and decreasing postprandially.[100] Ghrelin exerts its effects through a GH secretagogue receptor that is ubiquitously present in the body, indicating that it is associated with a variety of bodily functions.[99] Although ghrelin may have an adipogenic property, plasma ghrelin concentrations decrease with obesity in humans and dogs.[16,68,69,101,102] Weight reduction induced by energy restriction in obese humans and dogs has been reported to normalize plasma ghrelin concentrations.[16,68,103]

Decreased ghrelin concentrations may be caused by obesity-induced hyperleptinemia and hyperinsulinemia because they are inversely associated with plasma insulin and leptin concentrations in humans and dogs.[68,101,102] It is speculated that this suppression of ghrelin expression is an adaptive mechanism to the surplus of energy stores with obesity.[101] However, a reduced ability to decrease postprandial ghrelin concentrations in obese humans has been observed, which may explain hyperphagia even in a state of obesity.[76,102] Because exogenous ghrelin administration increased food intake of obese humans in a dose-dependent manner, its inhibition by leptin and insulin may be a more likely reason for continued hyperphagia than ghrelin resistance.[104]

Cholecystokinin (CCK) is secreted by I cells in the proximal small intestine and is known to promote nutrient digestion and to induce a negative feedback inhibition on appetite through the hypothalamus.[60,105] The major forms of plasma CCK include CCK8, CCK22, CCK33, and CCK58, which are denoted by different numbers of amino acids.[60] The data for CCK as it pertains to obesity is highly variable and contradictory. It was reported that obese women had greater fasting CCK concentrations than lean women, suggesting CCK's defensive action against overeating.[106] In contrast, one study showed markedly lower fasting and postprandial CCK concentrations in obese women as compared with lean women, indicating it as a reason for increased food intake with obesity.[102] There is also evidence that basal CCK concentrations are similar among nonobese, obese premenopausal, and postmenopausal women.[107] To our knowledge, no data are available on obese dogs and cats. Therefore, the effects of obesity on CCK regulation remain a question in humans and companion animals.

Glucagon-like peptide-1 (GLP-1) is produced by endocrine L cells in the distal small intestine and the large intestine.[105] The processing of preproglucagon by prohormone convertase 1 and 2 produces GLP-1, GLP-2, and oxyntomodulin, depending on the cleavage site.[105] GLP-1 is subsequently cleaved to form the biologically active peptides of GLP-1 (7–37) or GLP-1 (7–36) amide.[108] With the presence of nutrients in the small intestinal lumen, GLP-1 suppresses gastropancreatic secretion and gastric emptying under hypothalamic control and subsequently decreases food intake.[105] GLP-1 is also an "incretin" factor, stimulating insulin and inhibiting glucagon secretion after a meal.[105] A reduced postprandial GLP-1 response has been reported in obese as compared with lean humans.[109–112] Increased plasma glucose and free fatty acid concentrations, often a result of obesity, have been considered factors for blunted GLP-1 response with weight gain.[109,110] However, postprandial GLP-1, glucose, and free fatty acid concentrations have not been strongly correlated in obese

Table 1
Obesity-induced hormonal alterations in humans, dogs, and cats

Hormone	Humans	Dogs	Cats
Hypothalamus-pituitary axis			
Growth hormone	↓	ND	ND
IGF-1	↑, Normal, ↓	↑, Normal	ND
CRH, ACTH, cortisol	↑	↑, Normal	ND
TRH, TSH	↑, Normal, ↓	↑, Normal	Normal
T₃, T₄	↑, Normal	↑, Normal	Normal
Prolactin	↑, Normal	↑	↑
Total testosterone (male)	↓	↓	ND
Total testosterone (female)	↑	↑	ND
Estrogen	↑	ND	ND
Pancreas			
Insulin	↑	↑	↑
Glucagon	↑	ND	ND
Amylin	↑	ND	ND
Pancreatic polypeptide	↓	ND	ND
Adipose tissue			
Leptin	↑	↑	↑
Adiponectin	↓	↓	↓
Resistin	↑	ND	ND
TNF-α, IL-6	↑	↑	↑
Gastrointestinal tract			
Ghrelin	↓	↓	ND
Cholecystokinin	↑, Normal, ↓	ND	ND
Glucagon-like peptide-1	↓	↑	ND
Peptide YY	↓	ND	ND

Abbreviations: ACTH, corticotropin; CRH, corticotropin-releasing hormone; IGF-I, insulin-like growth factor-I; IL-6, interleukin-6; ND, no data available; T₃, triiodothyronine; T₄, thyroxine; TNF-α, tumor necrosis factor α; TRH, thyrotropin-releasing hormone; TSH, thyrotropin; ↑, increase; ↓, decrease.

humans.[111] In contrast to humans, one study reported a tendency for greater GLP-1 concentrations in obese than lean dogs.[16] However, no further data have been published to support this initial observation in dogs.

Peptide YY (PYY) is coproduced with GLP-1 by endocrine L cells in the distal small intestine and the large intestine. Two biologically active forms of PYY, PYY-1 (1–36) and PYY-2 (3–36), have been identified; PYY-2 is a predominant form in the circulation.[113] PYY and GLP-1 have very similar biologic functions, suggesting that these 2 hormones complement each other.[105] As observed in GLP-1 response, fasting and postprandial plasma PYY-2 concentrations have been reported to be lower in obese than in lean humans.[102,114] Postprandial plasma PYY-2 concentrations, which are typically increased in normal-weight subjects after a meal, were blunted in obese subjects.[102] This observation demonstrates that increased food intake with obesity may be partly a result of decreased plasma PYY concentrations.[102,105] However, obese humans showed no PYY resistance, as exogenous PYY infusion resulted in a similar reduction in caloric intake between obese and lean humans.[114] To our knowledge, the effect of obesity on PYY has not been examined in dogs and cats.

SUMMARY

Obesity is believed to induce various endocrine alterations and is characterized by blunted responsiveness to stimuli and hormonal resistance. Many of these alterations not only occur during the development of obesity but also modify metabolic systems that promote further weight gain and/or disease. Obesity-associated endocrine alterations are presented in **Table 1**, although the results are still inconclusive in many areas. Most abnormal hormone concentrations are corrected by weight reduction, which implicates obesity as a direct cause of the endocrine alterations. Several physiologic factors, including age, sex, puberty, and health status of obese subjects complicate the relationship between obesity and endocrine alterations. Significant hormone-hormone interactions, which were highlighted throughout the review, further complicate our understanding of their role in normal and obese states. It is clear, however, that a considerable amount of crosstalk occurs within and between tissues. Thus, research using whole animals must be sustained to fully understand these complicated systems. There has been a lack of published data pertaining to hormonal functions and the effects of obesity in dogs and cats. It may be conceivable that obesity-related hormonal alterations observed in humans are comparable to those of dogs and cats, but future research is required to verify this assumption.

REFERENCES

1. Sikaris KA. The clinical biochemistry of obesity. Clin Biochem Rev 2004;25(3): 165–81.
2. Lund EM, Amstrong PJ, Kirk CA, et al. Prevalence and risk factors for obesity in adult cats from private US veterinary practices. Int J Appl Res Vet Med 2005; 3(2):88–96.
3. Lund EM, Amstrong PJ, Kirk CA, et al. Prevalence and risk factors for obesity in adult dogs from private US veterinary practices. Int J Appl Res Vet Med 2005; 4(2):177–86.
4. Laflamme DP. Understanding and managing obesity in dogs and cats. Vet Clin North Am Small Anim Pract 2006;36(6):1283–95.
5. Scott-Moncrieff JC. Clinical signs and concurrent diseases of hypothyroidism in dogs and cats. Vet Clin North Am Small Anim Pract 2007;37(4):709–22.
6. Glass AR, Burman KD, Dahms WT, et al. Endocrine function in human obesity. Metabolism 1981;30(1):89–104.
7. Nam SY, Lee EJ, Kim KR, et al. Effect of obesity on total and free insulin-like growth factor (IGF)-1, and their relationship to IGF-binding protein (BP)-1, IGFBP-2, IGFBP-3, insulin, and growth hormone. Int J Obes 1997;21(5):355–9.
8. Luque RM, Kineman RD. Impact of obesity on the growth hormone axis: evidence for a direct inhibitory effect of hyperinsulinemia on pituitary function. Endocrinology 2006;147(6):2754–63.
9. Rasmussen MH, Hvidberg A, Juul A, et al. Massive weight loss restores 24 hour growth hormone release profiles and serum insulin-like growth factor-I concentrations in obese subjects. J Clin Endocrinol Metab 1995;80(4):1407–15.
10. Scacchi M, Pincelli AI, Cavagnini F. Growth hormone in obesity. Int J Obes 1999; 23(3):260–71.

11. Lee EJ, Kim KR, Lee HC, et al. Acipimox potentiates growth hormone response to growth hormone-releasing hormone by decreasing serum free fatty acid levels in hyperthyroidism. Metabolism 1995;44(11):1509–12.
12. Kratzsch J, Dehmel B, Pulzer F, et al. Increased serum GHBP levels in obese pubertal children and adolescents: relationship to body composition, leptin and indicators of metabolic disturbances. Int J Obes 1997;21(12):1130–6.
13. Douyon L, Schteingart DE. Effect of obesity and starvation on thyroid hormone, growth hormone, and cortisol secretion. Endocrinol Metab Clin North Am 2002;31(1):173–89.
14. Argente J, Caballo N, Barrios V, et al. Multiple endocrine abnormalities of the growth hormone and insulin-like growth factor axis in prepubertal children with exogenous obesity: effect of short- and long-term weight reduction. J Clin Endocrinol Metab 1997;82(7):2076–83.
15. Gayet C, Bailhache E, Dumon H, et al. Insulin resistance and changes in plasma concentration of TNF, IGF-1, and NEFA in dogs during weight gain and obesity. J Anim Physiol Anim Nutr 2004;88(3):157–65.
16. Yamka RM, Friesen KG, Frantz NZ. Identification of canine markers related to obesity and the effects of weight loss on the markers of interest. Int J Appl Res Vet Med 2006;4(4):282–92.
17. Martin LJM, Siliart B, Dumon HJW, et al. Hormonal disturbance associated with obesity in dogs. J Anim Physiol Anim Nutr 2006;90(9):355–60.
18. Guillaume-Gentil C, Rohner-Jeanrenaud F, Abramo F, et al. Abnormal regulation of the hypothalamo-pituitary-adrenal axis in the genetically obese fa/fa rat. Endocrinology 1990;126(4):1873–9.
19. Vicennati V, Ceroni L, Genghini S, et al. Sex difference in the relationship between the hypothalamic-pituitary-adrenal axis and sex hormones in obesity. Obesity (Silver Spring) 2006;14(2):235–43.
20. Roelfsema F, Kok P, Frolich M, et al. Disordered and increased adrenocorticotropin secretion with diminished adrenocorticotropin potency in obese premenopausal women. J Clin Endocrinol Metab 2009;94(8):2991–7.
21. Pasquali R, Cantobelli S, Casimirri F, et al. The hypothalamic-pituitary-adrenal axis in obese women with different patterns of body fat distribution. J Clin Endocrinol Metab 1993;77(2):341–6.
22. Fox CS, Pencina MJ, D'Agostino RB, et al. Relations of thyroid function to body weight: cross-sectional and longitudinal observations in a community-based sample. Arch Intern Med 2008;168(6):587–92.
23. Roti E, Minelli R, Salvi M. Thyroid hormone metabolism in obesity. Int J Obes Relat Metab Disord 2000;24(Suppl 2):S113–5.
24. Kokkoris P, Pi-Sunyer FX. Obesity and endocrine disease. Endocrinol Metab Clin North Am 2003;32(4):895–914.
25. Daminet S, Jeusette I, Duchateau L, et al. Evaluation of thyroid function in obese dogs and in dogs undergoing a weight loss protocol. J Vet Med A Physiol Pathol Clin Med 2003;50(4):213–8.
26. Ferguson DC, Caffall Z, Hoenig M. Obesity increases free thyroxine proportionally to nonesterified fatty acid concentrations in adult neutered female cats. J Endocrinol 2007;194(2):267–73.
27. Pinkney JH, Goodrick SJ, Katz J, et al. Leptin and the pituitary-thyroid axis: a comparative study in lean, obese, hypothyroid and hyperthyroid subjects. Clin Endocrinol 1998;49(5):583–8.

28. Reinehr T, Andler W. Thyroid hormones before and after weight loss in obesity. Arch Dis Child 2002;87(4):320–3.
29. Feldt-Rasmussen U. Thyroid and leptin. Thyroid 2007;17(5):413–9.
30. Kok P, Roelfsema F, Frölich M, et al. Prolactin release is enhanced in proportion to excess visceral fat in obese women. J Clin Endocrinol Metab 2004;89(9): 4445–9.
31. Doknic M, Pekic S, Zarkovic M, et al. Dopaminergic tone and obesity: an insight from prolactinomas treated with bromocriptine. Eur J Endocrinol 2002;147(1): 77–84.
32. Kopelman PG. Physiopathology of prolactin secretion in obesity. Int J Obes Relat Metab Disord 2000;24(Suppl 2):S104–8.
33. Donders SH, Pieters GF, Heevel JG, et al. Disparity of thyrotropin (TSH) and prolactin responses to TSH-releasing hormone in obesity. J Clin Endocrinol Metab 1985;61(1):56–9.
34. Lala VR, Ray A, Jamias P, et al. Prolactin and thyroid status in prepubertal children with mild to moderate obesity. J Am Coll Nutr 1988;7(5):361–6.
35. Martin LJ, Siliart B, Dumon HJ, et al. Spontaneous hormonal variations in male cats following gonadectomy. J Feline Med Surg 2006;8(5):309–14.
36. Pasquali R, Patton L, Gambineri A. Obesity and infertility. Curr Opin Endocrinol Diabetes Obes 2007;14(6):482–7.
37. Kyrou I, Tsigo C. Chronic stress, visceral obesity and gonadal dysfunction. Hormones 2008;7(4):287–93.
38. Vermeulen A, Kaufman JM, Deslypere JP, et al. Attenuated luteinizing hormone (LH) pulse amplitude but normal LH pulse frequency, and its relation to plasma androgens in hypogonadism of obese men. J Clin Endocrinol Metab 1993;76(5): 1140–6.
39. Ivandić A, Prpić-Krizevac I, Sucić M, et al. Hyperinsulinemia and sex hormones in healthy premenopausal women: relative contribution of obesity, obesity type, and duration of obesity. Metabolism 1998;47(1):13–9.
40. Smith SR. The endocrinology of obesity. Endocrinol Metab Clin North Am 1996; 25(4):921–42.
41. Beijerink NJ, Buijtels JJ, Okkens AC, et al. Basal and GnRH-induced secretion of FSH and LH in anestrous versus ovariectomized bitches. Theriogenology 2007;67(5):1039–45.
42. Günzel-Apel AR, Seefeldt A, Eschricht FM, et al. Effects of gonadectomy on prolactin and LH secretion and the pituitary-thyroid axis in male dogs. Theriogenology 2009;71(5):746–53.
43. Hoenig M. Comparative aspects of diabetes mellitus in dogs and cats. Mol Cell Endocrinol 2002;197(1–2):221–9.
44. Appleton DJ, Rand JS, Sunvold GD. Insulin sensitivity decreases with obesity, and lean cats with low insulin sensitivity are at greatest risk of glucose intolerance with weight gain. J Feline Med Surg 2001;3(4):211–28.
45. Fettman MJ, Stanton CA, Banks LL, et al. Effects of weight gain and loss on metabolic rate, glucose tolerance, and serum lipids in domestic cats. Res Vet Sci 1998;64(1):11–6.
46. Hoenig M, Thomaseth K, Waldron M, et al. Insulin sensitivity, fat distribution, and adipocytokine response to different diets in lean and obese cats before and after weight loss. Am J Physiol Regul Integr Comp Physiol 2007;292(1):R227–34.
47. Bergman RN, Kim SP, Hsu IR, et al. Abdominal obesity: role in the pathophysiology of metabolic disease and cardiovascular risk. Am J Med 2007;120(Suppl 1):S3–8.

48. Rand JS, Fleeman LM, Farrow HA, et al. Canine and feline diabetes mellitus: nature or nurture? J Nutr 2004;134(Suppl 8):S2072–80.
49. Ellmerer M, Hamilton-Wessler M, Kim SP, et al. Reduced access to insulin-sensitive tissues in dogs with obesity secondary to increased fat intake. Diabetes 2006;55(6):1769–75.
50. Houseknecht KL, Baile CA, Matteri RL, et al. The biology of leptin: a review. J Anim Sci 1998;76(5):1405–20.
51. Serisier S, Gayet C, Leray V, et al. Hypertriglyceridaemic insulin-resistant obese dog model: effects of high-fat diet depending on age. J Anim Physiol Anim Nutr 2008;92(4):419–25.
52. Malewiak MI, Griglio S, Kalopissis AD, et al. Oleate metabolism in isolated hepatocytes from lean and obese Zucker rats. Influence of a high fat diet and in vitro response to glucagon. Metabolism 1983;32(7):661–8.
53. Starke AA, Erhardt G, Berger M, et al. Elevated pancreatic glucagon in obesity. Diabetes 1984;33(3):277–80.
54. Solerte SB, Rondanelli M, Giacchero R, et al. Serum glucagon concentration and hyperinsulinaemia influence renal haemodynamics and urinary protein loss in normotensive patients with central obesity. Int J Obes Relat Metab Disord 1999;23(9):997–1003.
55. Young A. Inhibition of glucagon secretion. Adv Pharmacol 2005;52:151–71.
56. Reda TK, Geliebter A, Pi-Sunyer FX. Amylin, food intake, and obesity. Obes Res 2002;10(10):1087–91.
57. Reinehr T, de Sousa G, Niklowitz P, et al. Amylin and its relation to insulin and lipids in obese children before and after weight loss. Obesity (Silver Spring) 2007;15(8):2006–11.
58. O'Brien TD. Pathogenesis of feline diabetes mellitus. Mol Cell Endocrinol 2002; 197(1–2):213–9.
59. Lutz TA, Rand JS. Pathogenesis of feline diabetes mellitus. Vet Clin North Am Small Anim Pract 1995;25(3):527–52.
60. Hameed S, Dhillo WS, Bloom SR. Gut hormones and appetite control. Oral Dis 2009;15(1):18–26.
61. Lassmann V, Vague P, Vialettes B, et al. Low plasma levels of pancreatic polypeptide in obesity. Diabetes 1980;29(6):428–30.
62. Lieverse RJ, Masclee AA, Jansen JB, et al. Plasma cholecystokinin and pancreatic polypeptide secretion in response to bombesin, meal ingestion and modified sham feeding in lean and obese persons. Int J Obes Relat Metab Disord 1994;18(2):123–7.
63. Reinehr T, Enriori PJ, Harz K, et al. Pancreatic polypeptide in obese children before and after weight loss. Int J Obes 2006;30(10):1476–81.
64. Glaser B, Zoghlin G, Pienta K, et al. Pancreatic polypeptide response to secretin in obesity: effects of glucose intolerance. Horm Metab Res 1988; 20(5):288–92.
65. Lassmann V, Cabrerizzo GL, Vialettes B, et al. Impaired pancreatic polypeptide response to insulin hypoglycemia in obese subjects. Horm Metab Res 1985; 17(12):663–6.
66. Radin MJ, Sharkey LC, Holycross BJ. Adipokines: a review of biological and analytical principles and an update in dogs, cats, and horses. Vet Clin Pathol 2009;38(2):1–21.
67. Friedman JM, Halaas JL. Leptin and the regulation of body weight in mammals. Nature 1998;395(22):763–70.

68. Jeusette IC, Detilleux J, Shibata H, et al. Effects of chronic obesity and weight loss on plasma ghrelin and leptin concentrations in dogs. Res Vet Sci 2005; 79(2):169–75.
69. Jeusette IC, Lhoest ET, Istasse LP, et al. Influence of obesity on plasma lipid and lipoprotein concentrations in dogs. Am J Vet Res 2005;66(1):81–6.
70. Ishioka K, Soliman MM, Sagawa M, et al. Experimental and clinical studies on plasma leptin in obese dogs. J Vet Med Sci 2002;64(4):349–53.
71. Ishioka K, Hosoya K, Kitagawa H, et al. Plasma leptin concentration in dogs: effects of body condition score, age, gender and breeds. Res Vet Sci 2007; 82(1):11–5.
72. Sagawa MM, Nakadomo F, Honjoh T, et al. Correlation between plasma leptin concentration and body fat content in dogs. Am J Vet Res 2002;63(1):7–10.
73. Nishii N, Nodake H, Takasu M, et al. Postprandial changes in leptin concentrations of cerebrospinal fluid in dogs during development of obesity. Am J Vet Res 2006;67(12):2006–11.
74. Halaas JL, Gajiwala KS, Maffei M, et al. Weight-reducing effects of the plasma protein encoded by the obese gene. Science 1995;269(5223):543–6.
75. Scarpace PJ, Zhang Y. Leptin resistance: a predisposing factor for diet-induced obesity. Am J Physiol Regul Integr Comp Physiol 2009;296(3):R493–500.
76. English PJ, Ghatei MA, Malik IA, et al. Food fails to suppress ghrelin levels in obese humans. J Clin Endocrinol Metab 2002;87(6):2984–7.
77. Houseknecht KL, Mantzoros CS, Kuliawat R, et al. Evidence for leptin binding to proteins in serum of rodents and humans: modulation with obesity. Diabetes 1996;45(11):1638–43.
78. Hu E, Liang P, Spiegelman BM. AdipoQ is a novel adipose-specific gene dysregulated in obesity. J Biol Chem 1996;271(18):10697–703.
79. Ishioka K, Omachi A, Sagawa M, et al. Canine adiponectin: cDNA structure, mRNA expression in adipose tissues and reduced plasma levels in obesity. Res Vet Sci 2006;80(2):127–32.
80. Ishioka K, Omachi A, Sasaki N, et al. Feline adiponectin: molecular structures and plasma concentrations in obese cats. J Vet Med Sci 2009;71(2):189–94.
81. Yamauchi T, Kamon J, Waki H, et al. The fat-derived hormone adiponectin reverses insulin resistance associated with both lipoatrophy and obesity. Nat Med 2001;7(8):941–6.
82. Bastard JP, Maachi M, Lagathu C, et al. Recent advances in the relationship between obesity, inflammation, and insulin resistance. Eur Cytokine Netw 2006;17(1):4–12.
83. Gayet C, Leray V, Saito M, et al. The effects of obesity-associated insulin resistance on mRNA expression of peroxisome proliferator-activated receptor-gamma target genes, in dogs. Br J Nutr 2007;98(3):497–503.
84. Garaulet M, Hernández-Morante JJ, de Heredia FP, et al. Adiponectin, the controversial hormone. Public Health Nutr 2007;10(10A):1145–50.
85. Kadowaki T, Yamauchi T. Adiponectin and adiponectin receptors. Endocr Rev 2005;26(3):439–51.
86. Sinha MK, Songer T, Xiao Q, et al. Analytical validation and biological evaluation of a high molecular-weight adiponectin ELISA. Clin Chem 2007;53(12): 2144–51.
87. Schober F, Neumeier M, Weigert J, et al. Low molecular weight adiponectin negatively correlates with the waist circumference and monocytic IL-6 release. Biochem Biophys Res Commun 2007;361(4):968–73.

88. Rea R, Donnelly R. Resistin: an adipocyte-derived hormone. Has it a role in diabetes and obesity? Diabetes Obes Metab 2004;6(3):163–70.

89. Savage DB, Sewter CP, Klenk ES, et al. Resistin/Fizz3 expression in relation to obesity and peroxisome proliferator-activated receptor-gamma action in humans. Diabetes 2001;50(10):2199–202.

90. Steppan CM, Bailey ST, Bhat S, et al. The hormone resistin links obesity to diabetes. Nature 2001;409(6818):307–12.

91. Vozarova de Courten B, Degawa-Yamauchi M, Considine RV, et al. High serum resistin is associated with an increase in adiposity but not a worsening of insulin resistance in Pima Indians. Diabetes 2004;53(5):1279–84.

92. Weisberg SP, McCann D, Desai M, et al. Obesity is associated with macrophage accumulation in adipose tissue. J Clin Invest 2003;112(12):1796–808.

93. Coppack SW. Pro-inflammatory cytokines and adipose tissue. Proc Nutr Soc 2001;60(3):349–56.

94. Inadera H. The usefulness of circulating adipokine levels for the assessment of obesity-related health problems. Int J Med Sci 2008;5(5):248–62.

95. Miller C, Bartges J, Cornelius L, et al. Tumor necrosis factor-alpha levels in adipose tissue of lean and obese cats. J Nutr 1998;128(Suppl 12):S2751–2.

96. Hoenig M, McGoldrick JB, deBeer M, et al. Activity and tissue-specific expression of lipases and tumor-necrosis factor alpha in lean and obese cats. Domest Anim Endocrinol 2006;30(4):333–44.

97. Yudkin JS, Kumari M, Humphries SE, et al. Inflammation, obesity, stress and coronary heart disease: is interleukin-6 the link? Atherosclerosis 2000;148(2):209–14.

98. Sowers M, Jannausch M, Stein E, et al. C-reactive protein as a biomarker of emergent osteoarthritis. Osteoarthr Cartil 2002;10(8):595–601.

99. Muccioli G, Tschöp M, Papotti M, et al. Neuroendocrine and peripheral activities of ghrelin: implications in metabolism and obesity. Eur J Pharmacol 2002; 440(2-3):235–54.

100. Tschöp M, Weyer C, Tataranni PA, et al. Circulating ghrelin levels are decreased in human obesity. Diabetes 2001;50(4):707–9.

101. Zwirska-Korczala K, Konturek SJ, Sodowski M, et al. Basal and postprandial plasma levels of PYY, ghrelin, cholecystokinin, gastrin and insulin in women with moderate and morbid obesity and metabolic syndrome. J Physiol Pharmacol 2007;58(Suppl 1):13–35.

102. Konopko-Zubrzycka M, Baniukiewicz A, Wróblewski E, et al. The effect of intra-gastric balloon on plasma ghrelin, leptin, and adiponectin levels in patients with morbid obesity. J Clin Endocrinol Metab 2009;94(5):1644–9.

103. Cummings DE, Purnell JQ, Frayo RS, et al. A preprandial rise in plasma ghrelin levels suggests a role in meal initiation in humans. Diabetes 2001; 50(8):1714–9.

104. Druce MR, Wren AM, Park AJ, et al. Ghrelin increases food intake in obese as well as lean subjects. Int J Obes 2005;29(9):1130–6.

105. Huda MS, Wilding JP, Pinkney JH. Gut peptides and the regulation of appetite. Obes Rev 2006;7(2):163–82.

106. Baranowska B, Radzikowska M, Wasilewska-Dziubinska E, et al. Disturbed release of gastrointestinal peptides in anorexia nervosa and in obesity. Diabetes Obes Metab 2000;2(2):99–103.

107. Milewicz A, Bidzińska B, Mikulski E, et al. Influence of obesity and menopausal status on serum leptin, cholecystokinin, galanin and neuropeptide Y levels. Gynecol Endocrinol 2000;14(3):196–203.

108. Mojsov S, Kopczynski MG, Habener JF. Both amidated and nonamidated forms of glucagon-like peptide I are synthesized in the rat intestine and the pancreas. J Biol Chem 1990;265(14):8001–8.
109. Ranganath LR, Beety JM, Morgan LM, et al. Attenuated GLP-1 secretion in obesity: cause or consequence? Gut 1996;38(6):916–9.
110. Ranganath L, Norris F, Morgan L, et al. Inhibition of carbohydrate-mediated glucagon-like peptide-1 (7-36) amide secretion by circulating non-esterified fatty acids. Clin Sci 1999;96(4):335–42.
111. Verdich C, Toubro S, Buemann B, et al. The role of postprandial releases of insulin and incretin hormones in meal-induced satiety: effect of obesity and weight reduction. Int J Obes Relat Metab Disord 2001;25(8):1206–14.
112. Näslund E, Hellström PM. Glucagon-like peptide-1 in the pathogenesis of obesity. Drug News Perspect 1998;11(2):92–7.
113. Grandt D, Schimiczek M, Beglinger C, et al. Two molecular forms of peptide YY (PYY) are abundant in human blood: characterization of a radioimmunoassay recognizing PYY 1-36 and PYY 3-36. Regul Pept 1994;51(2):151–9.
114. Batterham RL, Cohen MA, Ellis SM, et al. Inhibition of food intake in obese subjects by peptide YY3-36. N Engl J Med 2003;349(10):926–8.

Obesity in Dogs and Cats: A Metabolic and Endocrine Disorder

Debra L. Zoran, DVM, PhD

KEYWORDS

- Obesity • Adipocytes • Adipokines • Leptin • Adiponectin
- Cytokines • Dog • Cat

Obesity is defined as an accumulation of excessive amounts of adipose tissue in the body, and has been called the most common nutritional disease of dogs in Western countries.[1–5] There have been a variety of surveys reporting the incidence of obesity in various parts of the world, and in these studies the incidence of obesity ranges from 22% to 44% depending on location and criteria.[5–9] However, in the past 10 years, most investigators have agreed that at least 33% of the dogs presented to veterinary clinics are obese, and that the incidence is increasing as human obesity increases in the overall population.[1] This statistic is important because obesity is not just the accumulation of large amounts of adipose tissue, but is associated with important metabolic and hormonal changes in the body. These metabolic and hormonal changes are the focus of this review, and are associated with a variety of conditions, including osteoarthritis, respiratory distress, glucose intolerance and diabetes mellitus, hypertension, dystocia, decreased heat tolerance, some forms of cancer, and increased risk of anesthetic and surgical complications.[1,6,10–14] Further, recent studies in a group of age-matched, pair-fed Labrador retrievers show that lean dogs have a significant increase in their median life span (of nearly 2.5 years) and a significant delay in the onset of signs of chronic disease.[15] Thus, prevention and early recognition of obesity, as well as correcting obesity when it is present, is essential to appropriate health care, and increases both the quality and quantity of life for pets.

The causes of obesity are multifactorial, and there are many genetic and environmental factors; however, obesity is ultimately related to energy imbalance: too many calories consumed or too few calories burned. Nevertheless, there is increasing evidence that outside factors play an important role in obesity development. One of these recognized factors is breed predisposition to obesity (likely a genetic factor, but this is unproven), and there are clearly other components, such as age, sex, gonadal status, and hormonal influences that play significant roles in the development of obesity. The dog breeds with increased risk of obesity are the Labrador retriever, Boxer,

Department of Small Animal Clinical Sciences, College of Veterinary Medicine and Biomedical Sciences, Texas A&M University, College Station, TX 77043-4474, USA
E-mail address: dzoran@cvm.tamu.edu

Vet Clin Small Anim 40 (2010) 221–239
doi:10.1016/j.cvsm.2009.10.009
0195-5616/10/$ – see front matter © 2010 Elsevier Inc. All rights reserved.

vetsmall.theclinics.com

Cairn terrier, Scottish terrier, Shetland sheepdog, Basset hound, Cavalier King Charles spaniel, Cocker spaniel, Dachshund (especially long-haired), Beagle, and some giant breed dogs.[3,6,16,17] However, some breeds are clearly resistant to development of obesity, with greyhounds being a notable example.[17] In addition to breed-related predisposition, obesity also tends to increase with age. This phenomenon is believed to result from the reduced metabolic rate that occurs with aging.[18] Further, Edney and Smith[6] reported a higher incidence of obesity in dogs with elderly owners, a phenomenon possibly related to food-, behavior-, and exercise-related factors. Obesity is more common in younger female dogs, but as both sexes reach old age (>12 years), 40% of both males and females are obese.[5,19–21] Another clear risk factor for obesity is neutering; the incidence of obesity is higher in neutered dogs of both sexes. This problem is believed to be due to hormonal changes associated with neutering and the reduced metabolic rate that occurs with the loss of sex hormones.[5,6,22] The reasons for this effect have been studied more in cats, but it is clear that sex hormones (and especially estrogen) are important regulators of energy intake and metabolism. Estrogen recently has been demonstrated to inhibit lipogenesis, and is known to be a determinant of adipocyte number.[23] Thus, changes in sex hormones following neutering seem to influence development of obesity by direct effects on the brain centers affecting satiety and metabolism (eg, the hypothalamus and others), and indirectly by affecting cell metabolism and hormonal regulators of food (eg, ghrelin and leptin).[17,24,25] The effect on energy metabolism is significant. A 30% decrease in energy intake was required to prevent post-spay weight gain in female Beagles.[25] In contrast, in a separate study of working dogs, increasing exercise after neutering also resulted in maintenance of ideal body condition compared with dogs that were not neutered.[26] Thus, either a reduction of intake by approximately one-third, or a proportionate increase in exercise, or a combination of both is required to prevent post-neuter weight gain in dogs. This early-age increase in body weight is a significant risk factor for adulthood obesity. As is the case in human childhood obesity, excess weight in puppyhood predisposes dogs to adult obesity, and obese females between 9 and 12 months of age are 1.5 times more likely to become obese as adults.[20] Similar kittenhood obesity study has not been reported in cats, but a similar phenomenon of weight gain following neutering does occur in young cats, predisposing them to early weight gains and the hormonal changes that come with it. Other important risk factors for obesity in dogs are endocrine disorders such as hypothyroidism and hyperadrenocorticism, medications that result in hyperphagia (anticonvulsants and glucocorticosteroids), consumption of table scraps, treats, free-choice feeding or poorly controlled meal feeding, high calorie home-cooked meals, and a sedentary lifestyle that results in a lack of significant exercise.[3,17,22]

The goal of the this review is to provide the reader an understanding of the importance of adipose tissue in normal metabolism, and especially in appetite, energy balance, and glucose and fat metabolism. In addition, the role of adipokines, hormones secreted from normal white adipose tissue, are reviewed in both the normal and obese state, giving the reader an insight into the important roles of these hormones in the body. There have been several recent reviews on the nutritional aspects of obesity and the important role of diet and exercise in the management of obesity, so the interested reader is referred to these articles for more information on this aspect of obesity management.[2,4,27]

THE ROLE OF ADIPOSE TISSUE IN NORMAL METABOLISM

Adipose tissue has traditionally been considered a diffuse, ill-defined tissue with the primary role of storing energy in the form of triglyceride, and a secondary role as insulation and protection for other body organs. In actuality, adipose tissue is a much more complex organ and contains a variety of cell types (**Fig. 1**). In adipose tissues, there are 2 types of adipocytes: white adipose tissue (WAT) and brown adipose tissue. WAT represents the majority of adipocytes in adult tissues and is the familiar image of fat tissue: many large triglyceride-filled cells surrounded by smaller cells and structures. The primary distinction between WAT and brown adipose is the presence of multilocular lipid droplets in brown fat that are actively involved in thermogenesis as a result of expression of distinct genes affecting mitochondrial function, including uncoupling protein-1, and that are found in higher proportions in neonates.[28,29] Adipose tissue is made up collectively of much more than adipocytes, which account for approximately 50% of the total cell population, but includes pre-adipocytes, multipotent mesenchymal stem cells, endothelial cells, pericytes, macrophages, and nerve cells.[30] The presence of stem cells and pre-adipocytes is crucial to the expansion of adipose tissue that occurs in obesity. These cells are recruited when existing adipocytes reach a critical level of hypertrophy, resulting in adipose tissue hyperplasia.[31] Monocytes and macrophages in adipose tissue have been identified as an important contributors to obesity-related disorders because they are sources of proinflammatory, procoagulant, and acute phase reactant cytokines (adipocytes and endothelial cells also produce these cytokines), and their numbers and activity increase as adipocytes hypertrophy.[28] In addition to understanding adipose tissue as a distinct organ with multiple cell types, research in rats, mice, and humans has shown that fat in different anatomic locations have distinct biologic behavior due to local influences in gene expression and differentiation.[32] In humans, it is clear that the pathologic sequelae of obesity are influenced by the preferential deposition of fat into visceral deposits instead of subcutaneous deposits (**Fig. 2**).[28,32] This phenomenon has been termed metabolic syndrome in humans, and is associated with abdominal obesity (accumulation of visceral adipose tissue), blood lipid disorders, inflammation, insulin resistance or type 2 diabetes, and increased risk of developing cardiovascular disease.[33,34] A difference in secretion of adipokines from regional adipose tissue sites similar to that reported in humans has been reported in cats and dogs,[35,36] but a true

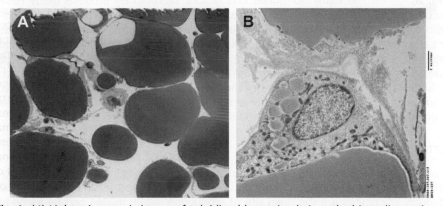

Fig. 1. (A) Light microscopic image of toluidine blue-stained visceral white adipose tissue. Small structures surrounding and interspersed between the triglyceride-filled adipocytes are primarily macrophages and vessels. (B) Electron micrograph of visceral white adipose tissue showing the ultrastructure of the nucleus of an adipocyte with multiple small fat-containing bodies, which are new adipocytes prior to being released. (*Courtesy of* Mr Ralph Nicholes and Dr Fred Clubb, Texas Heart Institute, Houston, TX.)

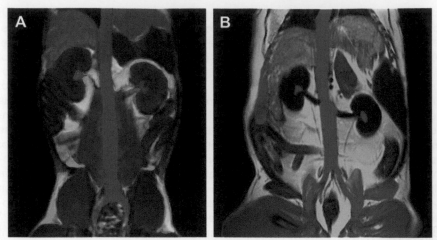

Fig. 2. (*A*) Magnetic resonance image (T1-weighted) of a normal dog (body condition score 4/9) illustrating the normal structures and small amount of intra-abdominal body fat. (*B*) Magnetic resonance image (T1-weighted) of an obese dog (body condition score 8/9) illustrating the large amounts of intra-abdominal fat. The image has been colorized to improved visualization of organs versus adipose. (*Courtesy of* Washington State University College of Veterinary Medicine, Pullman, WA; with permission.)

metabolic syndrome has not been described in these animals, likely, in part, due to differences in risk factors for cardiovascular disease and blood lipid abnormalities.

An important aspect of adipose tissue function was unknown until the mid-1990s with the discovery that WAT was the source of the hormone leptin. Since that time, WAT has become known as an important endocrine organ that secretes a wide variety of substances, including steroid hormones, growth factors and cytokines, eicosanoids, complement proteins, binding proteins, vasoactive factors, regulators of lipid and glucose metabolism, and others active in energy metabolism and appetite control (**Fig. 3**).[30,37–39] The many hormones and factors secreted by adipose tissue have become collectively known as adipokines. Adipokines are essential to normal physiologic function, and are important in the regulation of diverse biologic processes including energy balance, glucose and lipid metabolism, inflammation and immune function, hemostasis, vascular function, and angiogenesis.[30,40–42] There are more than 50 known adipokines. Of these, the most well known is leptin, but others, such as adiponectin, resistin, and some of the proinflammatory cytokines, for example, interleukins (IL), tumor necrosis factor alpha (TNFα), interferon gamma (IFNγ) and so forth, have been studied in multiple species, including dogs and cats.

LEPTIN

Leptin is the prototypical adipokine, and of all of the adipokines is the one best characterized in dogs and cats.[30,43–45] Leptin is a protein encoded by the *ob* gene, and although adipocytes are the main site of production, leptin mRNA can be found in placenta, mammary gland and liver in humans and rodents.[45] Although leptin is secreted constitutively by adipocytes, increased secretion is based on the energy flux within these cells, and circulating concentrations of leptin correlate with fat mass.[46] This correlation is true in all species examined to date, including dogs and cats.[35,36,47] Transcription of the *ob* gene and secretion of leptin are also controlled by

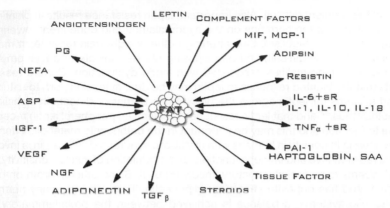

Fig. 3. Illustration of white adipose tissue (WAT) adipocytes showing and some of the hormones and cytokines secreted by this tissue. This illustration is not representative of all adipocytokines known to be produced by WAT. ASP, acylation stimulating protein; IGF, insulin-like growth factor; MCP, monocyte chemotactic protein; MIF, macrophage inhibitory factor; NGF, nerve growth factor; PAI, platelet activator inhibitor; PG, prostaglandin; sR, serine receptor; SAA, serum amyloid A; TGF, tumor growth factor; VEGF, vascular endothelial growth factor. (Illustration by Mr Larry Wadsworth, Texas A&M University, College Station, TX.)

a variety of metabolic and inflammatory mediators, including insulin, glucocorticoids, endotoxin, and such cytokines as TNFα, IL1β, and IL-6.[30,45] The effects of leptin are initiated, as with many adipokines, through interaction with its receptor. The leptin receptor family (Ob-R) is very closely related to members of the IL-6 family of receptors, and although the highest numbers of receptors are expressed in the satiety centers of the hypothalamus, they can be found widely distributed throughout the body, reflecting leptin's involvement in the regulation of diverse physiologic processes.[48–50]

When leptin, which is from the Greek "leptos" for thinness, was discovered, its primary actions were believed to be suppression of appetite and increased energy expenditure (via thermogenesis).[37,45,49] These early reports were based on mouse models showing that absence of leptin resulted in severe obesity.[51] Subsequent studies have shown that leptin binding to its receptor in the hypothalamus results in a series of events leading to suppression of appetite, including stimulation of anorexigenic neurons via neurotransmitters such as cocaine- and amphetamine-regulated transcript (CART), and melanocyte-stimulating hormone (MSH), suppression of orexigenic neurons (via neurotransmitters such as neuropeptide Y and agouti-related peptide), and suppression of the release of endocannabinoids, which are regulators of orexigenic neurons.[52–54] Although it is clear that leptin deficiency (either due to lack of the hormone or its receptor) results in development of severe obesity in rodents and humans, it is not a common cause of obesity in humans and has not been documented to date in dogs or cats.[55] Rather, the majority of obese humans, and dogs and cats as well, have high circulating concentrations of leptin, and the problem is not leptin deficiency but diminished end-organ response to leptin in the hypothalamus. Thus, obesity unrelated to specific genetic mutations in leptin or its receptor is characterized by leptin resistance and hyperleptinemia. Of note, hyperleptinemia in humans can also occur as a consequence of aging (independent of or disproportional to increases in body fat mass), but this phenomenon has not yet been reported in dogs or cats.[56,57] Unfortunately, the causes of leptin resistance are likely multifactorial, which make identification and reversal of the problem difficult. Also important, leptin resistance results in blunting of the satiety effects of the hormone on the hypothalamus and concurrent lowering of the body's energy metabolism, thus abetting further weight gain (or at least making weight loss extremely difficult) and predisposing obese subjects to development of other metabolic abnormalities associated with leptin dysfunction. Current research suggests that the blunted response to leptin may be due, at least in part, to saturated transport systems for leptin across the blood-brain barrier or defects in signaling in the hypothalamus,[42] and that leptin resistance is selective: peripheral leptin receptors continue to function and this may be important in the pathogenic metabolic effects of hyperleptinemia in obesity in humans with metabolic syndrome.[58,59] Leptin is involved in normal reproductive and immune function, and modulation of insulin sensitivity, and generally seems to be proinflammatory (mediated by IL-6 and others), prothrombotic, prooxidant, and has opposite effects to adiponectin. Thus, as with many hormonal and metabolic systems, a balance is achieved between the proinflammatory and anti-inflammatory effects of 2 hormones produced in adipocytes, leptin and adiponectin, and when the balance is disrupted due to development of obesity, it results in hyperleptinemia, leptin resistance, and development of obesity-related disorders.

Leptin in Dogs and Cats

Circulating concentrations of leptin correlate with fat mass in both dogs and cats.[60–66] Thus, increased fat mass, from either experimentally induced obesity or in pet dogs and cats with increased body condition scores, results in predictable, measurable increases in leptin. In contrast, reduction in fat mass also results in a decrease in leptin concentrations in both species.[35,61] There is ob gene expression in dog pre-adipocytes and mature adipocytes from WAT from multiple sites, but no expression in tissues other than WAT—a finding that has only been observed in the dog.[67] Studies of ob gene expression have not been reported in cats. In both dogs and cats, leptin concentrations are increased after a fatty or high-energy meal. In dogs, this effect can result in 2- to 3-fold increases of leptin concentrations for as long as 8 hours.[68] Of note, in cats the postprandial effect of dietary composition on leptin concentration is not consistent, but seems to be modulated by the relative insulin resistance and body fat mass.[69,70] Regardless of body condition score and fat mass, cats with insulin resistance (either due to diet or other causes) have higher circulating concentrations of leptin than cats with normal sensitivity to insulin.[71] Thus, the role of leptin in feline metabolism is clearly linked to insulin sensitivity and glucose metabolism. The issue of breed-related influences on metabolism and obesity is unsettled, primarily due to a paucity of published studies; however, results of a recent study by Ishioka and colleagues,[62] show that the breed of dog may influence leptin concentrations. For example, when examined within body condition score groups, Shetland sheepdogs had higher circulating leptin concentrations, whereas dachshunds, Shih Tzu, and Labrador retrievers had lower concentrations.[62] No specific breed-related studies on leptin have been reported in cats. Another factor affecting leptin concentrations in dogs is glucocorticosteroid therapy (eg, dexamethasone increases leptin concentrations in dogs, but prednisone seems to have no effect), and this may also influence feeding status, energy regulation, and other aspects of metabolism.[60,72] Finally, the effect of neutering on body weight and leptin status in cats has been a topic of considerable interest. In general, increases in leptin occur after neutering in cats, and are correlated with the amount of body fat gained post-neuter, and this effect occurs in both males and females.[65,73,74] The increases in leptin likely reflects the strong tendency for cats to gain weight post-neuter if their food intake is not closely regulated. Further studies are required to assess the role of neutering on body fat in cats.

ADIPONECTIN

After leptin, the next most studied and well-understood adipokine is adiponectin. When adiponectin was discovered (after the discovery of leptin in the mid-1990s), a variety of different names were ascribed, including Acrp 30, GBP28, and AdipoQ.[75] Unlike leptin, adiponectin is produced exclusively by mature adipocytes, after which it circulates as trimers, hexamers, or even high molecular weight multimers in very high concentrations. Adiponectin is among the most highly expressed genes in adipose tissue.[75] Adiponectin secretion is stimulated by insulin as well as by several drugs (eg, thiazolidinediones, and cannabinoid-1 receptor antagonists such as rimonabant) and dietary constituents (eg, fish oil, linoleic acid, soy protein).[76-78] These effects have not yet been reported in dogs or cats. Nevertheless, the role of adiponectin is tightly connected to glucose metabolism through enhancing insulin sensitivity and increasing glucose uptake via the GLUT 4 transporter.[79-81] In addition, adiponectin increases glycolysis by phosphorylation of phosphofructokinase and increases fatty acid oxidation, 2 functions that also are essential to enhanced glucose uptake and metabolism.[81] In humans, other well-characterized effects of include its anti-inflammatory properties (which are opposite of leptin) and inhibition of the development of atherosclerosis.[82] The beneficial cardiovascular effects of adiponectin may stem from its function as a vasodilator, an effect mediated through adiponectin's promotion of increased expression of endothelial nitric oxide synthase (iNOS) and prostacyclin synthase.[83,84] The anti-inflammatory effects of adiponectin seem to be due to the ability of the hormone to suppress TNFα production by macrophages.[85] Although these effects are being widely studied in humans, there are no reports yet in dogs or cats confirming similar physiologic effects in these species.

In the obese state, leptin concentrations are typically dramatically increased, reflecting the large increases in fat mass and leptin secretion. However, unlike leptin, increases in fat mass result in decreased concentrations of circulating adiponectin, and conversely, weight loss results in a return to normal adiponectin concentrations.[86] Furthermore, in humans adiponectin concentrations are negatively correlated with body fat mass, fasting insulin concentrations, and plasma triglyceride concentrations.[87] The mechanisms underlying this decrease in adiponectin are unknown, but changes seem to occur at 3 levels: decreased total adiponectin production (which is greatest with visceral adiposity), changes in relative proportions of the molecular weight forms of adiponectin (fewer high molecular weight forms are present in obese individuals), and changes in the expression of adiponectin genes (proinflammatory cytokines IL-6 and TNFα in the enlarging fat mass are inhibitors of these genes).[30,88] In humans, decreased circulating levels of adiponectin are linked to development of type 2 diabetes, insulin resistance, hypertension, and development of progressive ventricular hypertrophy,[89,90] and although these syndromes are commonly associated with obesity, the persistent reduction in adiponectin concentrations present even in persons matched for body mass and adiposity suggests that low circulating adiponectin concentration is an independent risk factor for development of metabolic complications.

Adiponectin in Dogs and Cats

Adiponectin nucleotide and amino acid sequences have been determined in both dogs and cats, and show strong homology to those of other species,[91-93] while canine adiponectin appears to circulate as variably sized complexes similar to human adiponectin. As in humans, both canine and feline adiponectin is highly expressed in WAT, and in cats the gene is expressed in significantly greater amounts in visceral adipose sites.[93] Similar to humans, both dogs and cats have lower circulating concentrations of adiponectin with increased fat mass, and in dogs the gene expression is also decreased (this is not yet been studied in cats).[35,47,92] Studies in dogs and cats indicate that adiponectin is predictably decreased in the obese state, suggesting that this hormone may have similar roles in the development of the metabolic changes, insulin resistance, and type 2 diabetes. Further work is needed to define the role of adiponectin in the development of feline diabetes, the incidence of which has greatly increased in recent years.

RESISTIN

Resistin was originally discovered as an adipokine secreted by murine adipocytes. This hormone is also found in human adipocytes, as well as in adipose tissues of cattle and pigs.[94–96] To date, expression of resistin has not been documented in dog or cat adipocytes, but the technical issues of assay development have been profound, and this may have slowed this discovery. In addition, the resistin receptor has also not yet been found. Thus, a great deal of work is needed to further define the presence and role of this adipokine in domestic animals and humans. However, the secretion of this hormone in rodents seems to follow leptin: circulating concentrations increase with increasing fat mass and following a meal. Hyperresistinemia results in development of insulin resistance and metabolic derangements typical of type 2 diabetes.[97,98] Increased concentrations of resistin are associated with proinflammatory cytokine secretion by macrophages, and in humans, increased resistin concentrations are correlated with atherosclerosis.[99] Additional work is required to fully understand the role of this adipokine in obesity-related disorders, especially those associated with dysregulation of glucose and development of insulin resistance.

ANGIOTENSINOGEN AND THE RENIN-ANGIOTENSIN-ALDOSTERONE SYSTEM

One of the best known metabolic/regulatory systems in the body is the renin-angiotensin-aldosterone system (RAAS), and its importance in vascular homeostasis, water balance, and renal function is well documented. Thus, the recognition that RAAS plays an important role in normal adipocyte biology, and particularly in adipocyte differentiation and metabolism, was a crucial discovery.[30] WAT is a major source of angiotensinogen in humans and rodents, second only to the liver in concentrations of this precursor to angiotensin II.[100] In fact, renin and angiotensin-converting enzyme are present in high concentrations in fat as well, and the local production of angiotensin II in adipose tissue seems to play a role in normal adipocyte differentiation, size, and insulin sensitivity.[100,101] In obese humans, increased production of angiotensinogen is a major contributor to the development of cardiovascular and kidney disease. Increases in angiotensinogen from adipocytes result in increased circulating concentrations of angiotensin II, which promotes increased vasoconstrictor activity (which can lead to hypertension or renal dysfunction), and increased concentrations of aldosterone, which promotes renal sodium retention.[100–102] Studies in obese rodents show that dysregulation of the RAAS system ultimately leads to reduced renal blood flow and glomerular filtration as well as to development of hypertension, both potentially very harmful to kidney function and development of renal disease.[100–102] As with resistin, the role of the RAAS system in adipocytes and in obesity in dogs and cats is not well understood. Only one study has documented the activation of the RAAS in diet-induced obesity in dogs, and in that study the focus was on the effects of RAAS activation on functional and structural changes in the kidney as a model of human disease.[102] Based on the importance of RAAS in obesity-associated diseases in humans and rodents, the role of RAAS in obese dogs and cats may also be important.

INFLAMMATORY CYTOKINES (INTERLEUKINS, TNFα, CHEMOTACTIC AND COMPLEMENT PROTEINS)

Obesity is considered to be a chronic inflammatory disease. In humans, the inflammation associated with obesity is known to cause insulin resistance, dyslipidemia (increased plasma triglycerides, decreases in high-density lipoprotein [HDL]-cholesterol, increases in low-density lipoprotein [LDL]-cholesterol), heart diseases (including atherosclerosis, hypertrophic cardiomyopathy, and heart failure secondary to the increased preload and afterload as a result of hypertension and fat mass), increased risk of hypertension and stroke, and osteoarthritis.[103–106] In normal-weight individuals, concentrations of proinflammatory cytokines secreted by adipose tissues are low or undetectable. However, in obesity, adipokine production is dysregulated, resulting in increased production of proinflammatory cytokines, while increased numbers of macrophages, which also secrete cytokines that promote the inflammatory process, are recruited to adipose tissue.[103] Although a wide variety inflammatory cytokines are produced by adipose tissue, TNFα and IL6 are the most widely studied cytokines produced by adipose tissue in any species, including dogs and cats.[30,39] TNFα was originally named for its ability to induce the necrosis of cancers after acute bacterial infection. However, this cytokine is actively involved in many processes, including inflammation, autoimmune diseases, tumorigenesis, viral replication, septic shock, fever, and obesity.[39,105,106] TNFα was first shown to be involved in adipocyte metabolism by suppressing the expression of many adiposespecific genes, such as lipoprotein lipase, and by stimulating lipolysis.[107] More recently, TNFα was found to have an important role in the development of insulin resistance as a result of its ability to downregulate GLUT 4 in adipose tissue.[108] Subsequent studies in rodents have proven a role of TNFα in the development of insulin resistance, but human studies attempting to neutralize the effects of the cytokine have shown less compelling improvements in insulin sensitivity. Thus, the complete role of this cytokine in the development of insulin resistance remains to be discovered. The interleukins, and specifically IL6, seem to have a significant role in obesity-associated inflammation in all species studied to date. In humans, serum concentrations of IL-6 are increased in type 2 diabetes and in metabolic syndrome, and correlate with an increase in body fat mass.[39] Some of the effects of IL-6 secreted from adipocytes include stimulation of hepatic triglyceride secretion, inhibition of insulin signaling in hepatocytes, and induction of hepatic C-reactive protein synthesis.[28,39] WAT is also a source of a variety of other inflammatory cytokines, including IFN-γ, other interleukins (IL-1, -8, -10, -18), C-reactive protein, monocyte chemotactic protein-1, and complement proteins, such as platelet activator inhibitor-1, Factor VII, and tissue factor (see **Fig. 2**).[28,37,39,109,110] In short, the chronic, subacute state of inflammation that accompanies the accumulation of WAT has been documented by the increases in circulating concentrations of inflammatory markers, and is further evidence that obesity-induced inflammation plays an important pathogenic role in the development and progression of obesity-related disorders.

INFLAMMATORY ADIPOKINES IN DOGS AND CATS

Studies in dogs have only recently begun to document the role of proinflammatory cytokines in the pathogenesis of obesity and obesity-related disorders in this species. Using reverse transcription-polymerase chain reaction to detect the mRNA of adipokines in dog adipocytes, investigators have detected genes for angiotensinogen, plasminogen activator inhibitor-1, IL-6, haptoglobin, metallothionein-1 and -2, and nerve growth factor in adipocytes of WAT.[37] Other investigators, in a study of experimentally induced obesity in dogs, reported increases in TNFα, insulin-like growth factor, and nonesterified fatty acids that were found concurrently with increased body fat mass and decreased insulin sensitivity.[47] Both of these studies mirror results in human and rodent studies, and suggest that obesity in dogs has many of the same physiologic and pathologic characteristics previously described in these species. Another study in obese dogs found that although the dogs developed biochemical evidence of insulin resistance, instead of having increased concentrations of C-reactive protein, concentrations were decreased significantly. This finding contrasts with those of studies in humans in which C-reactive protein concentrations increase in obesity.[111] Finally, studies of proinflammatory cytokines in feline obesity are lacking.

UNDERSTANDING OBESITY AS A DISEASE

Obese humans generally do not live as long as their lean counterparts, and are much more likely to suffer from obesity-related diseases.[112–114] Dogs and cats are susceptible to the same detrimental effects, including decreased longevity, and development of a variety of disorders that are also associated with human obesity (**Box 1**).[1] Dietary calorie restriction to maintain a lean body condition significantly increased longevity in a group of 24 Labrador retrievers.[15] In that study, the dogs in the energy-restricted group were fed approximately 25% less than their pair-fed counterparts (another group of 24 dogs), which were allowed to become overweight or obese. The lean dogs lived an average of 2 years longer than their overweight counterparts, and had reduced incidences of hip dysplasia, osteoarthritis, and glucose intolerance as well. This study and others illustrate that obesity is clearly associated with increased morbidity (in this study morbidity was associated with osteoarthritis) and early mortality.[11,15,115] Heat intolerance, increased anesthetic risk, increased difficulty with routine clinical procedures (catheter placement, palpation, imaging), and prolonged surgical procedures have also been documented in obese dogs.[1,27] Until recently, however, there were few studies in dogs, and even fewer in cats, that illustrated the increased disease risk associated with obesity.

As in humans, obesity in dogs and cats is associated with a variety of endocrine abnormalities. The most widely recognized and studied example is insulin resistance and the increased risk of development of type 2 diabetes.[35,47] The problem of obesity-induced insulin resistance is increasing in cats concurrent with the increase in type 2 diabetes in cats over the past 10 years.[71] In dogs, however, subclinical glucose intolerance and insulin resistance is often present without overt signs of diabetes. In addition to the hormonal effects of obesity on insulin function, there is an increasing body of evidence showing that obesity has a profound effect on thyroid hormone function. In one study, 42% of obese dogs had biochemical evidence of hypothyroidism (low serum free T_4 (fT4) concentrations, high serum thyrotropin [TSH] concentrations, or both), and of these dogs, a large percentage had no other clinical signs of hypothyroidism (similar to a phenomenon in humans termed subclinical hypothyroidism, in which TSH is increased and T_4 is either normal or decreased).[76] However, in an earlier study assessing the role of thyroid hormone in canine obesity, the only differences observed were in total T_4 and total T_3 concentrations, which were higher in the obese dogs.[116] This may occur as a result of thyroid hormone resistance, but no studies support this. Of note, in a study of obese cats, fT_4 concentrations increased significantly (some increases were within the normal range), and the increase was proportional to the increase in nonesterified fatty acids (NEFAs) (free fatty acids increase in feline obesity), a finding that may indicate that thyroid hormone uptake at the cellular level is inhibited by the presence of high concentrations of NEFAs.[117] Further clarification of the effects of obesity on thyroid hormone function is needed before specific

Box 1
Disorders associated with obesity

Orthopedic disorders

Osteoarthritis

Fractures (primarily humeral condyles)

Cruciate ligament tears/rupture

Intervertebral disk disease

Joint disorders

Endocrine and metabolic disorders

Hyperadrenocorticism

Hypothyroidism

Diabetes mellitus

Hypopituitarism

Hyperlipidemia

Glucose intolerance

Hepatic lipidosis (cats)

Cardiac and respiratory disorders

Pickwickian syndrome

Tracheal collapse

Laryngeal paralysis

Brachycephalic airway syndrome

Reduced airway compliance

Urogenital disorders

Urolithiasis (calcium oxalate)

Urethral sphincter mechanism incompetence

Transitional cell carcinoma

Mammary neoplasia

Dystocia

Idiopathic cystitis

Other miscellaneous disorders

Heat intolerance

Exercise intolerance

Increased anesthetic risk

Reduced life span

recommendations can be made; however, obesity seems to have a significant influence on thyroid hormones and their cellular function.

Dyslipidemias (alterations in cholesterol, triglycerides, and NEFAs) are commonly associated with obesity in humans, and in fact are one of the components of the metabolic syndrome. To date, only a few studies have been performed in either dogs or cats that further define changes in serum lipids in these species. However, one cross-sectional study in dogs evaluated the effect of obesity on serum concentrations of glucose, cholesterol, HDL-cholesterol, triglyceride, and on alanine aminotransferase activity, and found that significant increases in serum triglycerides and total cholesterol occurred in obese dogs.[118] These findings were confirmed in another clinical study assessing the utility of a bioelectric impedance device for assessment of body fat in dogs. In that study, serum cholesterol and triglyceride concentrations were also significantly higher in obese dogs than in lean dogs.[119] Another study of cats fed to achieve long-term obesity revealed similar changes in plasma lipids similar to those seen in obese people. Obese cats had increased NEFAs and triglycerides, decreased HDL, increased LDL, and overall increases in total cholesterol, and these changes occurred irrespective of diet.[120] In both dogs and cats, obesity seems to cause significant changes in lipid and lipoprotein metabolism that may be important in the development of other obesity-associated diseases.

Obese humans are prone to development of a variety of respiratory syndromes and airway distress, ranging from increased episodes of asthma to difficulty breathing due to Pickwickian-type obstruction of thoracic movement.[121,122] Few reports of similar conditions have appeared that address the effects of obesity on respiratory function in dogs or cats. However, there have been widespread anecdotal reports of obesity creating greater distress for dogs with tracheal collapse, laryngeal paralysis, and cats with asthma, suggesting a possible association. More evidence of the deleterious effects of obesity on the respiratory system have recently begun to surface, with the observations that obesity causes expiratory airway dysfunction in dogs.[14] In that study, normal breathing was unaffected by body condition, but in obese dogs (body condition score 9/9) during hyperpnea, expiratory airway resistance was markedly greater, indicating a dynamic flow limitation in these dogs that likely occurs in the distal airways.[14] No other abnormalities in airway function were observed. Further studies are needed to determine whether these changes are due to increases in inflammatory cytokines from obesity or due to airway wall resistance from decreased compliance. In either case, this study demonstrates that airway dysfunction, though subclinical in the majority of dogs, can occur. Studies of respiratory function in obese cats have not been published.

TREATMENT OF OBESITY

The management of obesity in dogs has long been focused on reducing energy consumption (dietary management) and increasing energy expenditure (exercise). This therapeutic approach is very effective when it is implemented completely and early[2,4]; however, it can be quite difficult to overcome the behavioral, social, metabolic, and hormonal influences of obesity in many dogs and cats. In humans, obesity management options include dietary management, exercise, behavior modification, pharmacologic therapy, and surgery. At this point, surgical therapy for obesity in dogs and cats has not been reported. For cats, there are currently no safe pharmacologic treatments for obesity, and until recently the options for dogs were limited to those products that reduced intestinal absorption of fat—a less than ideal approach with a significant therapeutic downside—and drugs that increased sympathetic tone, and were generally ineffective or potentially harmful.[3]

Dirlotapide (Slentrol) is a newer drug that is effective in treatment of obesity in dogs. The drug is a selective (intestinal) microsomal triglyceride transfer protein (MTP) inhibitor.[123] Dirlotapide reduces the absorption of fat from the small intestine by slowing the packaging of fatty acids and protein into chylomicrons, a process driven by MTP activity in the cytoplasm of the enterocyte. As a result of MTP inhibition, there is a reduction in fat absorption from the small intestinal lumen, but this is responsible for only a small fraction (approximately 10%) of the effect of dirlotapide on weight loss.[124] Further, because the fat is absorbed into the enterocyte, steatorrhea and other side effects related to fat malabsorption are minimal. Intracellular accumulation of fat due to MTP inhibition triggers release of peptide YY from the enterocyte into the systemic circulation.[124] Peptide YY is a potent appetite suppressant and satiety hormone, and is one of the peripheral hormones responsible for signaling the hypothalamus and other brain centers to control intake. The primary effect of dirlotapide is reduction in appetite. In clinical trials and in client-owned dogs, dirlotapide typically a causes reduction in food intake of about 10%.[123] The key benefit of adding dirlotapide to a weight loss program is that it influences one of the major obstacles to successful weight loss: it helps to control food intake. And although it is important to recognize that successful management of obesity requires appropriate dietary and exercise regimens, dirlotapide can be an effective tool in to the treatment of obesity.

SUMMARY

Obesity is the most common nutritional disorder of dogs and cats in Western countries. Although obesity is caused by an imbalance between energy intake and energy expenditure, there are many factors, both environmental and genetic, that influence this balance. Further, the alarming increase in obesity is important because this condition is associated with important metabolic and hormonal changes in the body. The systemic metabolic and hormonal changes that occur in obesity are the result of dysregulation of the adipokines secreted by WAT, and are the key factors in many diseases and disorders associated with obesity. The list of conditions associated with obesity is increasing as new research identifies the relationships between proinflammatory adipokines and disorders such as osteoarthritis, respiratory distress, diabetes mellitus, hypertension, dystocia, heat intolerance, and some forms of cancer. Because of the seriousness of obesity as a metabolic, hormonal, and inflammatory disease, prevention and management of obesity is essential.

REFERENCES

1. German AJ. The growing problem of obesity in dogs and cats. J Nutr 2006;136: 1940S–6S.
2. German AJ, Holden SL, Bissot T, et al. Dietary energy restriction and successful weight loss in obese client-owned dogs. J Vet Intern Med 2007;21:1174–80.
3. Gosselin J, Wren JA, Sunderland SL. Canine obesity: an overview. J Vet Pharmacol Ther 2007;30(Suppl 1):1–10.
4. Laflamme DP. Understanding and managing obesity in dogs and cats. Vet Clin North Am Small Anim Pract 2006;36:1283–95.
5. McGreevy PD, Thomson PC, Pride C, et al. Prevalence of obesity in dogs examined by Australian veterinary practices and the risk factors involved. Vet Rec 2005;156:696–707.
6. Edney AT, Smith PM. Study of obesity in dogs visiting veterinary practices in the United Kingdom. Vet Rec 1986;118:391–6.
7. Crane SW. Occurrence and management of obesity in companion animals. J Small Anim Pract 1991;32:275–82.
8. Kronfeld DS, Donoghue S, Glickman LT. Body condition and energy intakes of dogs in a referral teaching hospital. J Nutr 1991;121(Suppl 11):S157–8.

9. Lund EM, Armstrong PJ, Kirk CK, et al. Health status and population characteristics of dogs and cats examined at private veterinary practices in the United States. J Am Vet Med Assoc 1999;214:1336–41.
10. Fettman MJ, Stanton CA, Banks I, et al. Effects of neutering on body weight, metabolic rate and glucose tolerance in domestic cats. Res Vet Sci 1997;62: 131–6.
11. Kealy RD, Lawler DF, Ballam JM, et al. Evaluation of the effect of limited food consumption on radiographic evidence of osteoarthritis in dogs. J Am Vet Med Assoc 2000;217:1678–80.
12. Burkholder WJ. Precision and practicality of methods assessing body composition of dogs and cats. Comp Cont Ed Pract Vet 2001;23:1–10.
13. Montoya JA, Morris PJ, Bautista I, et al. Hypertension: a risk factor associated with weight status in dogs. J Nutr 2006;136:2011S–3S.
14. Bach JF, Rozanski EA, Bedenice D, et al. Association of expiratory airway dysfunction with marked obesity in healthy dogs. Am J Vet Res 2007;68:670–5.
15. Kealy RD, Lawler DF, Ballam JM, et al. Effect of diet restriction on life span and age-related changes in dogs. J Am Vet Med Assoc 2002;220:1315–20.
16. Meyer H, Drochner W, Weidenhaupt C. [A contribution to the occurrence and treatment of obesity in dogs]. Dtsch Tierarztl Wochenschr 1978;85:133–6 [in German].
17. Diez M, Nguyen P. The epidemiology of canine and feline obesity. Waltham Focus 2006;16:2–8.
18. Robertson ID. The association of exercise, diet and other factors with owner perceived obesity in privately owned dogs from metropolitan Perth, WA. Prev Vet Med 2003;58:75–83.
19. Sloth C. Practical management of obesity in dogs and cats. J Small Anim Pract 1992;33:178–82.
20. Glickman LT, Sonnenschein EG, Goickman NW, et al. Pattern of diet and obesity in female adult pet dogs. Vet Clin Nutr 1995;2:6–13.
21. Armstrong PJ, Lund EM. Changes in body composition and energy balance with aging. Vet Clin Nutr 1996;3:83–7.
22. Jeusette I, Detilleaux J, Cuvelier C, et al. Ad libitum feeding following ovariectomy in female Beagle dogs: effect on maintenance energy requirement and on blood metabolites. J Anim Physiol Anim Nutr 2004;88:117–21.
23. Cooke PS, Naaz A. Role of estrogens in adipocyte development and function. Exp Biol Med 2004;229:1127–35.
24. Houpt KA, Hintz HF. Obesity in dogs. Canine Pract 1978;5:54–8.
25. Jeusette I, Lhoest ET, Istasse L, et al. Influence of obesity on plasma lipid and lipoprotein concentrations in dogs. Am J Vet Res 2007;68.
26. LeRoux PH. Thyroid status, oestradiol level, work performance and body mass of ovariectomised bitches. J S Afr Vet Assoc 1983;54:115–7.
27. Blanchard G, Nguyen P, Gayet C, et al. Rapid weight loss with a high-protein low-energy diet allows the recovery of ideal body composition and insulin sensitivity in obese dogs. J Nutr 2004;134:2148S–50S.
28. Lafontan M. Fat cells: afferent and efferent messages define new approaches to treat obesity. Annu Rev Pharmacol 2005;45:119–46.
29. Rousset S, Alves-Guerra MC, Mozo J, et al. The biology of mitochondrial uncoupling proteins. Diabetes 2004;53:S130–5.
30. Radin MJ, Sharkey LC, Holycross BJ. Adipokines: a review of biological and analytical principles and an update in dogs, cats, and horses. Vet Clin Pathol 2009;38:136–56.

31. Fischer-Posovaszky P, Wabistsch M, Hochberg Z. Endocrinology of adipose tissue—an update. Horm Metab Res 2007;39:314–21.
32. Wajchenberg BL. Subcutaneous and visceral adipose tissue: their relation to the metabolic syndrome. Endocr Rev 2000;21:697–738.
33. Despres JP, Lemieux I. Abdominal obesity and metabolic syndrome. Nature 2006;444:881–7.
34. Fernandez ML. The metabolic syndrome. Nutr Rev 2007;65:S30–4.
35. Hoenig M, Caffail Z, Ferguson DC. Triiodothyronine differentially regulates key metabolic factors in lean and obese cats. Domest Anim Endocrinol 2007;34:229–37.
36. Leray V, Serisier S, Khosniat S, et al. Adipose tissue gene expression in obese dogs after weight loss. J Anim Physiol Anim Nutr 2008;92:390–8.
37. Badman MK, Flier JS. The adipocytes as an active participant in energy balance and metabolism. Gastroenterologist 2007;132:2103–15.
38. Rosen ED, Spiegelman B. Adipocytes as regulators of energy balance and glucose homeostasis. Nature 2006;444:847–52.
39. Juge-Aubry CE, Henrichot E, Meier CA. Adipose tissue: a regulator of inflammation. Best Pract Res Clin Endocrinol Metab 2005;19:547–66.
40. Lago F, Dieguez C, Gomez-Reino J, et al. Adipokines as emerging mediators of immune response and inflammation. Nat Clin Pract Rheumatol 2007;3:716–24.
41. Goldstein BJ, Scalia R. Adiponectin: a novel adipokine linking adipocytes and vascular function. J Clin Endocrinol Metab 2004;89:2563–8.
42. Pan W, Kastin AJ. Adipokines and the blood brain barrier. Peptides 2007;28:1317–30.
43. Iwase M, Kimura K, Sasaki N, et al. Canine leptin: cDNA cloning, expression and activity of recombinant protein. Res Vet Sci 2000;68:109–14.
44. Sakaki N, Shibata H, Honjoh T, et al. cDNA cloning of feline leptin and its mRNA expression in adipose tissue. J Vet Med Sci 2001;63:1115–20.
45. Harris RBS. Leptin: much more than a satiety signal. Annu Rev Nutr 2000;20:45–75.
46. Considine RV, Sinha MK, Heiman ML, et al. Serum immunoreactive leptin concentrations in normal weight and obese humans. N Engl J Med 1996;334:292–5.
47. Gayet C, Baihache E, Dumon H, et al. Insulin resistance and changes in plasma concentrations of TNFα, IGF1, and NEFA in dogs during weight gain and obesity. J Anim Physiol Anim Nutr 2004;88:157-65.
48. Tartaglia LA, Dembski M, Weng X, et al. Identification and expression cloning of a leptin receptor, OB-R. Cell 1995;83:1263–71.
49. Houseknecht LK, Portocarrero CP. Leptin and its receptors: regulators of whole body energy homeostasis. Domest Anim Endocrinol 1998;15:457–75.
50. Baumann H, Morella KK, White DW, et al. The full-length leptin receptor has signaling capabilities of interleukin 6-type receptors. Proc Natl Acad Sci U S A 1996;93:8374–8.
51. Zhang Y, Proenca R, Maffei M, et al. Positional cloning of the mouse obese gene and its human homologue. Nature 1994;372:425–32.
52. Ahima RS, Prabakaran D, Mantzoros CS, et al. Role of leptin in the neuroendocrine response to fasting. Nature 1996;382:250–2.
53. Cowley MA, Smart JL, Rubinstein M, et al. Leptin activates anorexigenic POMC neurons through a neural network in the arcuate nucleus. Nature 2001;411:480–4.
54. Balthasar N, Coppari R, McMinn J, et al. The hypothalamic arcuate nucleus: a key site for mediating leptin's effects on glucose homeostasis and locomotor activity. Cell Metab 2005;1:63–72.

55. Farooqui IS, Wangensteen T, Collins S, et al. Clinical and molecular genetic spectrum of congential deficiency of the leptin receptor. N Engl J Med 2007; 356:237–47.
56. Gabriely N, Ma XH, Yang XM, et al. Removal of visceral fat prevents insulin resistance and glucose intolerance of aging. Diabetes 2002;51:2951–8.
57. Wang Y. Cross-national comparison of childhood obesity: the epidemic and the relationship between obesity and socioeconomic status. Int J Epidemiol 2001; 30:1129–36.
58. Margetic S, Gazzola C, Regg GG, et al. Leptin: a review of its peripheral actions and interactions. Int J Obes Relat Metab Disord 2002;26:1407–33.
59. Correia MLG, Rahmouni K. Role leptin in the cardiovascular and endocrine complications of metabolic syndrome. Diabetes Obes Metab 2006;8:603–10.
60. Ishioka K, Soliman MM, Sagawa M, et al. Experimental and clinical studies on plasma leptin in obese dogs. J Vet Med Sci 2002;64:349–53.
61. Jeusette IC, Lhoest ET, Istasse LP, et al. Influence of obesity on plasma lipid and lipoprotein concentrations in dogs. Am J Vet Res 2005;66:81–6.
62. Ishioka K, Hosoya K, Kitagawa H, et al. Plasma leptin concentration in dogs: effects of body condition score, age, gender, and breeds. Res Vet Sci 2007; 82:11–5.
63. Backus RC, Havel PJ, Gingerich RL, et al. Relationship between serum leptin immunoreactivity and body fat mass as estimated by use of a novel gas-phase Fourier transform infrared spectroscopy deuterium dilution method in cats. Am J Vet Res 2000;61:796–801.
64. Appleton DJ, Rand JS, Sunvold GD. Plasma leptin concentrations in cats: Reference range, effect of weight gain and relationship with adiposity as measured by dual energy x-ray absorptiometry. J Feline Med Surg 2000;2:191–9.
65. Martin L, Siliart B, Dumon H, et al. Leptin, body fat content and energy expenditure in intact and gonadectomized adult cats: a preliminary study. J Anim Physiol Anim Nutr 2001;85:195–9.
66. Hoenig M, Ferguson DC. Effects of neutering on hormonal concentrations and energy requirements in male and female cats. Am J Vet Res 2002;63:634–9.
67. Eisele I, Wood IS, German AJ, et al. Adipokine gene expression in dog adipose tissues and dog white adipocytes differentiated in primary culture. Horm Metab Res 2005;37:474–81.
68. Ishioka K, Hatai H, Komabayashi K, et al. Diurnal variations of serum leptin in dogs: effects of fasting and re-feeding. Vet J 2005;169:85–90.
69. Thiess S, Becskei C, Tomsa K, et al. Effects of high carbohydrate and high fat diet on plasma metabolite levels and on IV glucose tolerance test in intact and neutered male cats. J Feline Med Surg 2004;6:207–18.
70. Backus RC, Cave NJ, Keisler DH. Gonadectomy and high dietary fat but not high dietary carbohydrate induce gains in body weight and fat of domestic cats. Br J Nutr 2007;98:641–50.
71. Appleton DJ, Rand JS, Sunvold GD. Plasma leptin concentrations are independently associated with insulin sensitivity in lean and overweight cats. J Feline Med Surg 2002;4:83–93.
72. Nishii N, Takasu M, Ohba Y, et al. Effects of administration of glucocorticoids and feeding status on plasma leptin concentrations in dogs. Am J Vet Res 2006;67:266–70.
73. Belsito KR, Vester BM, Keel T, et al. Impact of ovariohysterectomy and food intake on body composition, physical activity, and adipose gene expression in cats. J Anim Sci 2009;87:594–602.

74. Martin LJM, Siliart B, Dumon H, et al. Spontaneous hormonal variations in male cats following gonadectomy. J Feline Med Surg 2006;8:309–14.

75. Kadowaki T, Yamauchi T. Adiponectin and adiponectin receptors. Endocr Rev 2005;26:439–51.

76. Bensaid M, Gary-Bobo M, Esclangon A, et al. The cannabinoid CB1 receptor antagonist SR141716 increases ACRP30 mRNA in adipose tissue of obese fa/fa rats and in cultured adipocytes cells. Mol Pharmacol 2003;63:908–14.

77. Rossi AS, Lombardo YB, Lacorte JM, et al. Dietary fish oil positively regulates plasma leptin and adiponectin levels in sucrose fed, insulin resistant rats. Am J Physiol Regul Integr Comp Physiol 2005;289:R486–94.

78. Nagasawa A, Fukui K, Kojima M, et al. Divergent effects of soy protein diet on the expression of adipocytokines. Biochem Biophys Res Commun 2003;311:909–14.

79. Pajvani UB, Du X, Combs TP, et al. Structure-function studies of the adipocyte-secreted hormone ACRP30-adiponectin. Implications for metabolic regulation and bioactivity. J Biol Chem 2003;278:9073–85.

80. Yamauchi T, Kamon J, Minokoshi Y, et al. Adiponectin stimulates glucose utilization and fatty acid oxidation by activating AMP activated protein kinase. Nat Med 2002;8:1288–95.

81. Kadowaki T, Yamauchi T, Kubota N, et al. Adiponectin and adiponectin receptors in insulin resistance, diabetes, and the metabolic syndrome. J Clin Invest 2006;116:1784–92.

82. Hopkins TA, Ouchi N, Shibata R, et al. Adiponectin actions in the cardiovascular system. Cardiovasc Res 2007;74:11–8.

83. Fesus G, Dubrovska G, Gorzelnaik K, et al. Adiponectin is a novel humoral vasodilator. Cardiovasc Res 2007;75:719–27.

84. Shibata R, Izumiya Y, Sato K, et al. Adiponectin protects against the development of systolic dysfunction following myocardial infarction. J Mol Cell Cardiol 2007;42:1065–74.

85. Yokota T, Oritani K, Takahashi I, et al. Adiponectin, a new member of the family of soluble defense collagens, negatively regulates the growth of myelomonocytic progenitors and the functions of macrophages. Blood 2000;96:1723–32.

86. Hu E, Liang P, Spiegelman BM. AdipoQ is a novel adipose-specific gene dysregulated in obesity. J Biol Chem 1996;271:10697–703.

87. Cnop M, Havel PJ, Utzschneider KM, et al. Relationship of adiponectin to body fat distribution, insulin sensitivity, and plasma lipoproteins: evidence of independent roles of age and sex. Diabetologia 2003;46:459–69.

88. Bruun JM, Lihn AS, Verdich C, et al. Regulation of adiponectin by adipose tissue-derived cytokines: in vivo and in vitro investigations in humans. Am J Physiol Endocrinol Metab 2003;285:E527–33.

89. Furukawa S, Fujita T, Shimabukuro M, et al. Increased oxidative stress in obesity and its impact on metabolic syndrome. J Clin Invest 2004;114:1752–61.

90. Hong SD, Park CG, Seo HS, et al. Associations among plasma adiponectin, hypertension, left ventricular diastolic dysfunction, and left ventricular mass index. Blood Press 2004;13:236–42.

91. Brunson BL, Zhong Q, Clarke KJ, et al. Serum concentrations of adiponectin and characterization of adiponectin protein complexes in dogs. Am J Vet Res 2007;68:57–62.

92. Ishioka K, Omachi A, Sagawa M, et al. Canine adiponectin: cDNA structure, mRNA expression adipose tissues and reduced plasma levels in obesity. Res Vet Sci 2006;80:127–32.

93. Zini E, Linscheid P, Franchini M, et al. Partial sequencing and expression of genes involved in glucose metabolism in adipose tissues and skeletal muscle of healthy cats. Vet J 2009;80:66–70.

94. Lazar MA. Resistin and obesity associated metabolic diseases. Horm Metab Res 2007;39:710–6.

95. Komatsu T, Itoh F, Mikawa S, et al. Gene expression of resistin in adipose tissue and mammary gland of lactating and non-lactating cows. J Endocrinol 2003; 178:R1–5.

96. Dai MH, Xia T, Chen XD, et al. Cloning and characterization of porcine resistin gene. Domest Anim Endocrinol 2006;30:88–97.

97. Banerjee RR, Rangwala SM, Shapiro JS, et al. Regulation of fasted blood glucose by resistin. Science 2004;303:1195–8.

98. Steppan C, Bailey ST, Bath S, et al. The hormone resistin links obesity to diabetes. Nature 2001;409:307–12.

99. Steppan CM, Lazar MA. The current biology of resistin. J Intern Med 2004;255: 439–47.

100. Engeli S, Schling P, Gorzelniak K, et al. The adipose tissue renin-angiotensin-aldosterone system: role in the metabolic syndrome. Int J Biochem Cell Biol 2003;35:807–25.

101. Rahmouni K, Mark AI, Haynes WG, et al. Adipose depot specific modulation of angiotensinogen gene expression in diet induced obesity. Am J Physiol Endocrinol Metab 2004;286:E891–5.

102. Henegar JR, Bigler SA, Henegar LK, et al. Functional and structural changes in the kidney in the early stages of obesity. J Am Soc Nephrol 2001;12:1211–7.

103. Lee YH, Pratley RE. The evolving role of inflammation in obesity and the metabolic syndrome. Cuurr Diab Rep 2005;5:70–5.

104. Greenberg AS, Obin MS. Obesity and the role of adipose tissue in inflammation and metabolism. Am J Clin Nutr 2006;83:461S 5S.

105. Wisse BE. The inflammatory syndrome: the role of adipose tissue cytokines in metabolic disorders linked to obesity. J Am Soc Nephrol 2004;15:2792–800.

106. Bastard JP, Maachi M, Lagathu C, et al. Recent advances in the relationship between obesity, inflammation and insulin resistance. Eur Cytokine Netw 2006;17:4–12.

107. Hotamisligil GS, Shargill NS, Speigelman BM. Adipose expression of tumor necrosis factor alpha: direct role in obesity linked insulin resistance. Science 1993;259:87–91.

108. Moller DE. Potential role of TNF alpha in the pathogenesis of insulin resistance and type 2 diabetes. Trends Endocrinol Metab 2000;11:212–7.

109. Hotamisligil GS. The role of TNF alpha and TNF receptors in obesity and insulin resistance. J Intern Med 2006;245:621–5.

110. Merlens I, Van Gaal LF. Visceral fat as a determinant of fibrinolysis and hemostasis. Semin Vasc Med 2005;5:48–55.

111. Veiga APM, Price CA, Oliveira ST, et al. Association of canine obesity with reduced serum levels of C-reactive protein. J Vet Diagn Invest 2008;20:224–8.

112. Kopelman PG. Obesity as a medical problem. Nature 2000;404:635–43.

113. Vega GL. Obesity and the metabolic syndrome. Minerva Endocrinol 2004;29: 47–54.

114. Trayhurn P, Beattie I. Physiological role of adipose tissue: white adipose tissue as an endocrine and secretory organ. Proc Nutr Soc 2001;60:329–39.

115. Smith GK, Mayhew PD, Kapatkin AS, et al. Evaluation of risk factors for degenerative joint disease in association with hip dysplasia in German shepherd dogs,

golden retrievers, Labrador retrievers, and Rottweilers. J Am Vet Med Assoc 2001;219:1719–24.

116. Daminet S, Jeusette I, Duchateau L, et al. Evaluation of thyroid function in obese dogs and in dogs undergoing a weight loss protocol. J Vet med A Physiol Pathol Clin Med 2003;50:213–8.

117. Ferguson DC, Caffail Z, Hoenig M. Obesity increases free thyroxine proportionally to nonesterified fatty acid concentrations in adult neutered female cats. J Endocrinol 2007;194:267–73.

118. Pena C, Suarez L, Bautista I, et al. Relationship between analytic values and canine obesity. J Anim Physiol Anim Nutr 2008;92:324–5.

119. Stone RC, Berghoff N, Steiner JM, et al. Use of a bioelectric impedance device in obese and lean healthy dogs to estimate body fat percentage. Vet Ther 2009; 10:1–12.

120. Jordan E, Kley S, Le NA, et al. Dyslipidemia in obese cats. Domest Anim Endocrinol 2008;35:290–9.

121. Sin DD, Sutherland ER. Obesity and the lung: obesity and asthma. Thorax 2008; 63:1018–23.

122. Johnston RA, Theman TA, Lu FL, et al. Diet induced obesity causes innate airway hyperresponsiveness to methacholine and enhances ozone-induced pulmonary inflammation. J Appl Physiol 2008;104:1727–35.

123. Wren JA, Gossellin J, Sunderland SJ. Dirlotapide: a review of its properties and role in the management of obesity in dogs. J Vet Pharmacol Ther 2007;30(Suppl 1):11–6.

124. Wren JA, King VL, Campbell SL, et al. Biologic activity of dirlotapide, a novel microsomal triglyceride transfer protein inhibitor, for weight loss in obese dogs. J Vet Pharmacol Ther 2007;30(Suppl 1):33–42.

Insulin Resistance in Cats

J. Catharine Scott-Moncrieff, MS, MA, Vet MB

KEYWORDS

• Insulin • Diabetes mellitus • Insulin resistance
• Hyperadrenocorticism • Acromegaly

Insulin resistance is defined as decreased sensitivity to insulin. Insulin resistance is an important component of the pathogenesis of type 2 diabetes mellitus (DM), and resolution of peripheral insulin resistance in cats with type 2 DM together with good glycemic control may result in diabetic remission. In insulin-dependent diabetic cats, insulin resistance is manifested clinically as an inadequate response to an appropriate pharmacologic dose of insulin. There is no specific insulin dose that is diagnostic for insulin resistance; however most diabetic cats can be controlled on insulin doses ranging from 1 to 3 U per dose (<1 U/kg).[1–5] Cats that require insulin doses higher than 6 U per dose (>1.5 U/kg) to achieve good glycemic control, cats that have persistent hyperglycemia despite this dose of insulin, and cats with insulin needs that fluctuate or increase significantly over time should be evaluated for insulin resistance. This article focuses on the clinical problem of insulin resistance in insulin-dependent diabetic cats.

PATHOPHYSIOLOGY OF FELINE DM

DM is a common endocrine disease in cats characterized by an absolute or relative deficiency of insulin. Type 1 DM (insulin-dependent DM) is characterized by beta cell loss and minimal secretory response to β-cell secretagogues. Type 2 DM (non-insulin-dependent DM) is characterized by abnormal insulin secretion in conjunction with peripheral insulin resistance. The two types of DM are classically distinguished by response to insulin secretagogues such as glucose, glucagon, or arginine. In type 1 DM, there is decreased or negligible secretion of insulin compared with normal animals, whereas in type 2 DM, total insulin secretion may be normal or increased, with an abnormal pattern of insulin secretion. Up to 80% of diabetic cats are believed to have type 2 DM at the time of diagnosis; however, this is

Department of Veterinary Clinical Sciences, Purdue University, VCS/LYNN, 625 Harrison Street, West Lafayette, IN 47907, USA
E-mail address: scottmon@purdue.edu

Vet Clin Small Anim 40 (2010) 241–257
doi:10.1016/j.cvsm.2009.10.007
0195-5616/10/$ – see front matter © 2010 Elsevier Inc. All rights reserved.

vetsmall.theclinics.com

a clinical estimate only, because differentiation of the two forms of DM is clinically challenging in cats.

PATHOGENESIS OF INSULIN RESISTANCE

The causes of insulin resistance are classified depending upon whether there is interference with the availability of insulin to bind with the insulin receptor (prereceptor), interference with binding of insulin to the receptor (receptor), or factors that influence signal transduction after the interaction of insulin with the receptor (postreceptor). Receptor and postreceptor causes are difficult to distinguish and often occur concurrently. Destruction of insulin after subcutaneous administration and binding of exogenous insulin by anti-insulin antibodies are potential causes of prereceptor problems; however, these problems have been documented rarely in cats. Poor absorption of insulin from the subcutaneous site has been postulated as the cause of a poor clinical response to ultralente insulin in some cats.[1] The most common causes of insulin resistance in cats are mediated by secretion of hormones that antagonize the effects of insulin due to receptor or postreceptor causes (**Table 1**). Glucocorticoids, progestagens, catecholamines, thyroid hormones, growth hormone, and glucagon are implicated most commonly. The role of sex hormones and androgens in insulin resistance is unknown. Stress hyperglycemia mediated by catecholamines is common in cats and may mimic insulin resistance.[6]

CLINICAL INDICATORS OF INSULIN RESISTANCE

Cats with clinically significant insulin resistance typically present with signs of poor glycemic control such as persistent polyuria, polydipsia, polyphagia, weight loss, and peripheral neuropathy despite insulin doses greater than 1.5 U/kg (6 U per dose). Specifically, clinical indications of poor glycemic control are recurrence or persistence of clinical signs of diabetes mellitus; clinical signs of hypoglycemia (lethargy, disorientation, seizures); insulin dose higher than 6 U per dose or 1.5 U/kg; and recurrent ketoacidosis.

Cats with insulin resistance usually have persistent hyperglycemia on blood glucose (BG) curves and increased serum fructosamine concentrations. Conversely, if the insulin dose has been increased inappropriately or if the severity of insulin resistance fluctuates, affected cats may have clinical signs of hypoglycemia such as disorientation or seizures. Insulin resistance must be differentiated from other causes of poor glycemic control. Specifically, causes of poor glycemic control in diabetic cats include problems with owner compliance; inappropriate insulin dose or formulation; insulin-induced hypoglycemia (Symogi effect); rapid metabolism of insulin; and insulin resistance.

Other differential diagnoses usually can be excluded by the history and evaluation of a BG curve.

CAUSES OF INSULIN RESISTANCE IN CATS

There are currently no published prospective or retrospective studies specifically evaluating the causes of insulin resistance in cats. Common concurrent diseases identified in cats with DM or diabetic ketoacidosis include pancreatitis, hepatic lipidosis, cholangiohepatitis, urinary tract infection, renal failure, hyperthyroidism, inflammatory bowel disease, acromegaly, and heart disease.[7–14] Treatment with exogenous glucocorticoids or progestagens is also a common historical finding. Clinical experience suggests that these concurrent problems also cause insulin resistance in cats

Table 1
Proposed mechanisms of hormone-mediated insulin resistance in cats

Hormone	Proposed Mechanism(s) of Insulin Resistance	Associated Disease States
Glucocorticoids	Increased hepatic gluconeogenesis Decreased tissue use of glucose Decreased receptor affinity for insulin Decreased number and affinity of glucose transporters Increased glucagon and free fatty acid concentrations	Stress Hyperadrenocorticism Exogenous administration
Progesterone, progestagens	Reduced insulin binding Reduced glucose transport in tissues	Diestrus/pregnancy Exogenous administration (eg, megestrol acetate) Progestagen-secreting adrenal tumors
Growth hormone	Decreased number of insulin receptors Inhibition of glucose transport Decreased glucose use Increased glucose production Postinsulin receptor defect in peripheral tissues Increased lipolysis	Acromegaly
Glucagon	Activation hepatic glycogenolysis Increased hepatic glucose production	Bacterial infection Pancreatitis Trauma Congestive heart failure Renal failure Glucagonoma
Thyroid hormones	Decreased insulin synthesis and secretion Impaired insulin receptor binding Postreceptor defect Disproportionate increase in proinsulin secretion	Hyperthyroidism
Epinephrine	Stimulation of hepatic and renal glucose production Decreased glucose use Decreased insulin secretion Stimulation of glucagon secretion Mobilization of gluconeogenic precursors	Stress Pheochromocytoma

(**Box 1**). In a study of 104 cats with DM, glycemic regulation was worse in 21 cats with concurrent disease than in 33 cats without concurrent disease.[11] The severity of insulin resistance varies with the underlying disease. In some disorders, the resistance can be overcome by increasing the dose or changing the insulin formulation to a more potent product. In other diseases such as acromegaly, insulin resistance is severe and cannot be overcome by even extremely large insulin doses.[14,15] Disorders such as chronic pancreatitis often cause fluctuating insulin resistance. The insulin requirement in these cases fluctuates with time and increasing the insulin dose may lead to intermittent hypoglycemia.

Obesity

Obesity causes insulin resistance in cats and is important in the pathogenesis of DM in cats. Obesity occurs when energy intake exceeds energy output, and risk factors in cats include excessive food intake, indoor confinement, and physical inactivity.[16] Insulin sensitivity decreases by more than 50% in obese compared with healthy weight cats.[17] Insulin resistance associated with obesity in diabetic cats is typically mild and reversible and can be overcome by relatively small increases in insulin dose. In addition, cats with poor glycemic control undergo significant weight loss, so obesity alone is rarely a cause of severe insulin resistance. Acromegalic cats usually have a stable weight or gain weight despite poor glycemic control, so acromegaly should be considered in obese cats with profound insulin resistance.

Exogenous Glucocorticoids or Progestagens

Exogenous glucocorticoids and progestagens such as megestrol acetate cause insulin resistance (see **Table 1**). Administration of these drugs has been identified as an important precipitating factor for DM in cats.[9,11] Use of these drugs in an established diabetic cat may cause clinically significant insulin resistance and should be

| Box 1 |
Causes of insulin resistance in cats
Drug administration (progestagens/corticosteroids)
Infection (urinary tract/oral cavity/sepsis)
Hyperthyroidism
Acromegaly
Pancreatitis
Renal disease
Hepatic disease
Cardiac insufficiency
Hyperlipidemia
Neoplasia
Severe obesity
Exocrine pancreatic insufficiency
Hyperadrenocorticism
Pheochromocytoma

avoided. In cats with DM that require treatment with either glucocorticoids or progestagens for concurrent disease, the dose should be reduced to the minimum that will control the disease process, and the insulin dose should be increased cautiously to control hyperglycemia.

Pancreatitis

Pancreatitis is a common and frustrating problem in cats and may contribute to the pathogenesis of feline DM. Pancreatitis is also a common concurrent disease in diabetic cats and an important cause of insulin resistance. In a report of 37 diabetic cats that underwent necropsy, acute or subacute pancreatitis was identified in 2 cats; chronic pancreatitis was identified in 17 cats, and pancreatic neoplasia was identified in 8 cats.[11] Chronic inflammation due to pancreatitis causes insulin resistance that may impair glycemic regulation (see **Table 1**). In a study of 104 cats with DM, there was a trend for poorer glycemic control in cats with pancreatitis compared with those without.[11] Compounding the problem of insulin resistance in cats with pancreatitis is the cyclic nature of the disease. Because both insulin demands and appetite fluctuate with the severity of inflammation, clinical signs of poor glycemic control often coexist with an increased risk of clinical hypoglycemia.

Diagnosis of pancreatitis relies on evaluation of clinical signs; physical examination; abdominal ultrasound; and measurement of serum lipase, feline trypsin-like immunoreactivity, or feline pancreatic lipase immunoreactivity.[18] Unfortunately, in some cats it may be difficult to confirm a diagnosis without resorting to exploratory laparotomy and histopathology. Treatment of chronic pancreatitis in cats relies on use of intravenous fluid therapy, nutritional support, antiemetics, analgesia, and sometimes-cautious use of glucocorticoids. In general, the long-term prognosis for resolution of pancreatic inflammation is guarded.

Bacterial Infection

Bacterial infection is an important cause of insulin resistance in diabetic patients (see **Table 1**). Hyperglucagonemia has been implicated as the cause of insulin resistance in people with bacterial infection, but this has yet to be documented in the cat. Cats with DM are at increased risk of bacterial infection, especially of the urinary tract. Decreased urine concentration and glucosuria increase the likelihood of bacterial proliferation within the urinary tract. In a study of 141 diabetic cats that underwent urine collection by cystocentesis, urinary tract infection was identified in 13% of cats.[12] Only 40% of the cats with urinary tract infections exhibited clinical signs. Other studies also have documented that bacterial infections are common concurrent diseases in diabetic cats.[7,11] Other common sites of bacterial infection include the oral cavity, the skin, and the biliary tract. Other factors that have been hypothesized to increase the risk of infection in patients with DM include impaired humoral and cell-mediated immunity, abnormal neutrophil chemotaxis, and defects in phagocytosis and intracellular killing of bacteria.[1]

Renal Disease

Renal disease is common in diabetic cats. and glomerulosclerosis is the most common histopathologic finding.[9,11] Renal insufficiency may occur secondary to DM (diabetic nephropathy) or be a concurrent disorder. Moderate to severe renal failure may cause insulin resistance; however, cats also may be at increased risk for hypoglycemia because of decreased renal clearance of insulin.[1] Thus patients with concurrent renal failure and DM may be frustrating to manage. Problems with glycemic regulation may be compounded by anorexia. Polyuria and polydipsia caused by renal failure make the assessment of glycemic regulation more challenging. Diagnosis of renal disease relies on evaluation of physical examination findings and review of the minimum database (complete blood cell count [CBC], serum chemistry profile, urinalysis). Diagnostic tests that are helpful in further evaluating the cause of renal dysfunction in diabetic cats include urine culture, measurement of urine protein:creatinine ratio, and ultrasound examination of the urinary tract.

Hyperthyroidism

Hyperthyroidism has been reported to cause insulin resistance in both experimental and naturally occurring hyperthyroidism. Hyperthyroid cats have normal resting BG and insulin concentrations but have abnormal glucose tolerance.[19,20] Surprisingly, insulin resistance in spontaneous hyperthyroidism did not resolve after resolution of hyperthyroidism, possibly because of the influence of obesity.[20] Because both DM and hyperthyroidism are common disorders in geriatric cats, evaluation of thyroid status should be included in the minimum database of all geriatric diabetic cats. The diagnosis of hyperthyroidism is usually straightforward and is based on history, physical examination, and documentation of increased serum concentration of total T4. Confirming a diagnosis of hyperthyroidism may be more challenging in cats with severe systemic illness because of the effect of concurrent disease on resting thyroid hormone concentrations.[21] Additional diagnostic tests that may be necessary in such cats include measurement of free T4, a T3 suppression test, or scintigraphy.

Heart Disease

Heart disease also may cause insulin resistance and predisposition to ketoacidosis in diabetic cats. In a retrospective study of 20 diabetic cats and 57 control cats in a primary care practice, cats with DM were 10 times more likely to die of heart failure than control cats.[10] Occult heart disease should be considered in any diabetic cat with unexplained insulin resistance. Diagnosis is made by evaluation of the history and physical examination, thoracic radiography, electrocardiography, and echocardiography.

Neoplasia

Underlying nonendocrine neoplasia such as lymphoma or mast cell tumor are also common concurrent disorders in diabetic cats and may contribute to insulin resistance.[7–9] The diagnosis usually is made by evaluation of the history, physical examination, clinicopathologic abnormalities, results of diagnostic imaging, and histopathology. Bone marrow aspiration and more advanced imaging may be required in some cases.

Acromegaly

Acromegaly is caused by excess secretion of growth hormone from a pituitary adenoma.[22–24] Excess circulating growth hormone (GH) causes insulin resistance, carbohydrate intolerance, hyperglycemia and DM (see **Table 1**). Excess GH results in increased secretion of insulin growth factor 1 (IGF-1) from the liver and peripheral tissues. The anabolic effects of IGF-1 cause proliferation of bone, cartilage, and soft tissues, with resultant organomegaly. Although feline acromegaly in the past was considered a rare disorder, recent studies suggest that it may be a more common cause of insulin resistance in diabetic cats than previously was recognized.[14,15,24] In a study of 184 diabetic cats with a wide range of glycemic control, 32% of cats had markedly increased IGF-1 concentrations, and acromegaly was confirmed in 17 of these cats.[14]

Most cats with acromegaly are middle-aged or older (median 10 years of age, range 4 to 17 years), and 90% are male (intact or castrated).[14,15,22–24] All reported cases to date have had DM at the time of diagnosis. Clinical signs include evidence of poor glycemic control (polyuria, polydipsia, and polyphagia), large body size, weight gain despite poor glycemic control, and enlargement of the head and extremities (**Fig. 1**). Respiratory stridor is reported in up to 53% of acromegalic cats and is caused by enlargement of the tongue and oropharyngeal tissues.[14] Acromegalic cats tolerate high doses of insulin. Median insulin dose in one group of 17 acromegalic cats was 7 U every 12 hours (range 2 to 35 U), and in another group of 19 acromegalic cats, the dose was 1.9 U/kg (range 1.1 to 4.3).[14,15] Physical examination may reveal abdominal organomegaly, inferior prognathia, cataracts, clubbed paws, broad facial features, widened interdental spaces, cardiac murmurs or arrhythmias, respiratory stridor, lameness, peripheral neuropathy, and central neurologic signs attributable to an enlarging pituitary mass (**Fig. 2**). Cardiomegaly and renomegaly may be evident on imaging studies. Although weight loss caused by poorly regulated DM may occur initially, a key finding in acromegalic cats is weight gain or a stable weight (lack of weight loss) in a diabetic cat that by all other indications has poor glycemic control. Many acromegalic cats have a high body weight (range 3.5 to 9 kg), but as a group the body weights of acromegalic cats are not significantly greater than those of diabetic cats without acromegaly.[14,15]

Some cats with acromegaly may be phenotypically indistinguishable from normal cats. Acromegaly therefore should be considered in the differential diagnosis of any cat with insulin resistance if other more common causes have been ruled out, especially if the body weight is stable to increasing. Some clinicians have recommended evaluation for acromegaly in any cat that does not go into diabetic remission with appropriate diet and insulin therapy.[24]

A tentative diagnosis of acromegaly is made by measurement of GH and IGF-1 concentrations, and assays for both IGF-1 and GH have been validated in the cat.[14,25–27] Measurement of IGF-1 is a good screening test for acromegaly and has a specificity of 92% and sensitivity of 84% in diabetic cats with insulin resistance.[15] IGF-1 concentrations may be low in untreated diabetic cats, while some poorly controlled diabetic cats have slightly increased IGF-1 concentrations.[25,27] GH concentration is increased in most acromegalic cats.[26] GH has a short half-life and is episodically secreted; this is likely why there is some overlap in GH concentrations with nonacromegalic diabetic cats.[27] Ideally, both IGF-1 and GH concentration should

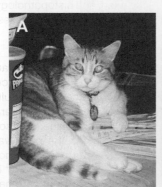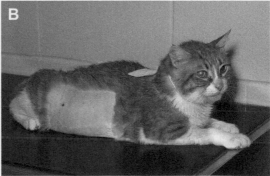

Fig. 1. Photograph of a 10-year-old male castrated cat three years before (*A*) and at time of diagnosis of (*B*) diagnosis of acromegaly.

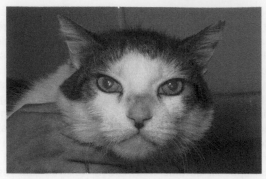

Fig. 2. Photograph of an 11-year male domestic short hair (DSH) cat with acromegaly demonstrating enlargement of the head and mild prognathia inferior.

be measured in a cat with suspected acromegaly. Imaging of the brain should be performed to confirm the diagnosis.[14,15] In most acromegalic cats, a pituitary tumor can be identified by either computed tomography (CT) or magnetic resonance imaging (MRI) (**Fig. 3**). In one case of confirmed acromegaly, acidophil proliferation within the pituitary gland did not result in a detectable mass on CT or MRI.[14] Thus even negative MRI findings do not preclude a diagnosis of acromegaly.

Radiation therapy is the most effective treatment for feline acromegaly. Radiation therapy has been reported to result in improvement of neurologic signs and decreased insulin requirements or diabetic remission in cats with acromegaly.[28–31] Interestingly, IGF concentrations do not decrease in concert with the clinical response.[30] Median survival in 14 cats treated with radiation therapy was 28 months.[30] Unfortunately, the cost and availability of radiation therapy often limit access to treatment.

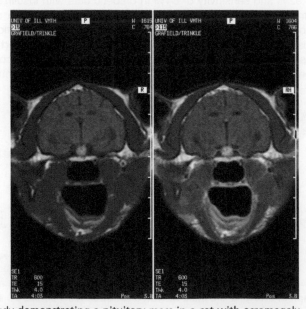

Fig. 3. MRI study demonstrating a pituitary mass in a cat with acromegaly.

Hypophysectomy has not been evaluated extensively in the treatment of feline acromegaly, although trans-sphenoidal cryohypophysectomy was used successfully to treat one acromegalic cat.[32] Neither octreotide nor L-deprenyl has been effective in amelioration of clinical signs of acromegaly in cats. In cats in which radiation therapy is not possible because of financial or logistical concerns, long-term survival may be achieved in acromegalic cats if DM is managed with high doses of insulin. Because of the profound insulin resistance associated with acromegaly, hypoglycemic complications using this approach are unusual. A median survival time of 20 months was reported in a group of 14 acromegalic cats, of which only 2 were treated with radiation and octreotide.[23] Cause of death in these cats was most commonly due to renal failure or congestive heart failure or a combination.[23]

Hyperadrenocorticism

Hyperadrenocorticism (HAC) is also an important cause of insulin resistance in cats. HAC is caused by excess secretion of adrenocortical hormones from either a functional pituitary tumor (PDH) or a functional tumor of the adrenal cortex. Cortisol is the most common hormone secreted in HAC; however, other adrenal hormones such as androstenedione, progesterone, 17- hydroxyprogesterone, estradiol, aldosterone and testosterone also may be secreted in cats with functional adrenocortical tumors. Eighty-five percent of cats with HAC have PDH, while 15% are diagnosed with functional adrenocortical tumors. Approximately 80% of cats with HAC are diabetic at the time of diagnosis.

Cats with HAC are middle aged to older (median 10 years of age, range 5 to 16 years), and females are slightly over-represented.[1,33–35] Clinical signs include evidence of poor glycemic control (polyuria, polydipsia, polyphagia, weight loss, and peripheral neuropathy), lethargy, abdominal enlargement or a pot-bellied appearance, muscle atrophy, unkempt hair coat, bilaterally symmetric alopecia, cutaneous fragility, and recurrent abscess formation (**Fig. 4**). Cats with HAC are predisposed to bacterial infection, so clinical signs of urinary tract infection, pyoderma and respiratory tract infection also may be present. Physical examination may reveal hepatomegaly, seborrhea, thinning of the skin, and cutaneous lacerations in addition to the clinical signs already discussed. Skin fragility may be so severe that tearing of the skin occurs during routine grooming of the hair coat (**Fig. 5**). Virilization caused by excess sex hormone secretion and hyperaldosteronism also have been reported in cats with HAC.[36,37] The results of a CBC, biochemical panel, and urinalysis are usually consistent with the presence of DM. Increased alkaline phosphatase, alanine transferase, hypercholesterolemia, hyperglycemia, and low serum urea nitrogen (BUN) are common. Cats do not have a steroid-induced isoenzyme of alkaline phosphatase, so changes in this enzyme are less prominent than seen in dogs, and increases likely are caused by poorly regulated DM. Endocrine tests used to confirm the diagnosis include the corticotropin (ACTH) stimulation test, the low-dose dexamethasone suppression test, and the urine cortisol:creatinine ratio (C:Cr). The urine cortisol:creatinine ratio is a useful screening test for hyperadrenocorticism.[38–41] Urine for measurement of the C:Cr ratio should be collected at home to minimize the influence of stress. If the C:Cr ratio is normal, HAC is unlikely; however, increases also may occur in cats with other concurrent illness, so additional testing is necessary for confirmation.[38] The low-dose dexamethasone suppression test is performed using a higher dose of dexamethasone (0.1 mg/kg intravenously) than in the dog. A baseline blood sample is collected, and additional samples are collected at 4 and 8 hours after dexamethasone administration. Serum cortisol concentration is suppressed (<1.5 µg/dL, <40 mmol/L) at 8 hours in normal cats but not in cats with HAC. A few cats with HAC will have

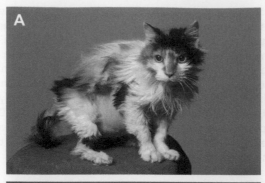

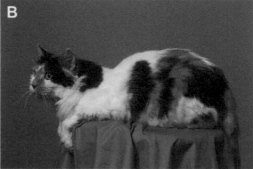

Fig. 4. (*A*) Photograph of a 14-year-old female spayed domestic long haired cat with pituitary-dependent hyperadrenocorticism. Note the unkempt hair coat, alopecia, muscle atrophy, and pot-bellied appearance. (*B*) Same cat after 6 months of treatment with trilostane at a dose of 25 mg by mouth every 12 hours.

a normal result with this dose of dexamethasone. If the index of suspicion for HAC is high, a second test using the lower dose of dexamethasone (0.01 mg/kg) can be performed. Interpretation is difficult, however, because serum cortisol concentrations in some normal cats will not be suppressed at this dose. The ACTH stimulation test is not a particularly sensitive or specific test in cats, but it is useful in cases in which dexamethasone suppression testing is difficult to interpret and in cats with suspected

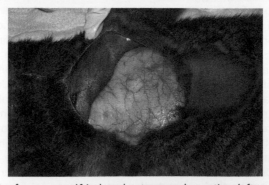

Fig. 5. Photograph of a severe self induced cutaneous laceration (after grooming) in a 12-year-old female spayed cat with hyperadrenocorticism.

iatrogenic HAC.[1] The ACTH stimulation test is performed using a dose of 125 μg of Cortrosyn administered intravenously or intramuscularly. Samples should be collected at baseline, and at 30 and 60 minutes after IM administration of ACTH, or 60 and 90 minutes after intravenous administration.[42] A post-ACTH serum cortisol concentration greater than 150 μg/dL (413 nmol/L) in a cat with clinical signs consistent is supportive of a diagnosis of HAC.[1,35,43]

Some adrenal carcinomas in cats have been associated with high circulating concentrations of other adrenal hormones such as androstenedione, progesterone, 17- hydroxyprogesterone estradiol, testosterone, and aldosterone (**Fig. 6**).[36,37,44,45] Cortisol concentrations in these cases are typically low, with little response to ACTH stimulation. A sex hormone-secreting tumor should be suspected in cats with clinical signs of HAC, an adrenal mass detected by ultrasound, and a blunted cortisol response to ACTH. All cats reported to date with sex hormone-secreting adrenal tumors have had adrenocortical carcinomas. Confirmation is by a sex hormone profile with hormones measured before and after ACTH stimulation testing.

Tests that are helpful for differentiation of pituitary-dependent from adrenal-dependent hyperadrenocorticism in cats include the high-dose dexamethasone suppression test (0.1 mg/kg or 1 mg/kg intravenously), endogenous ACTH stimulation, and abdominal ultrasonography.[1,41] Unfortunately, there is little published information comparing the diagnostic performance of these tests in cats. Clinical experience suggests that

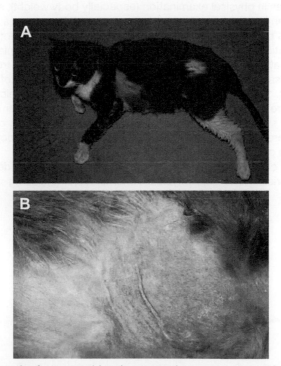

Fig. 6. (*A*) Photograph of a 7-year-old male castrated DSH cat with a sex hormone-secreting adrenal tumor. Note the unkempt hair coat and the areas of alopecia at the locations of previous cutaneous laceration. (*B*) Close-up view of the skin in the same cat showing severe thinning of the skin.

measurement of endogenous ACTH and adrenal ultrasonography are the most reliable differentiating tests.[41,46]

Treatment options for cats with HAC depend upon whether the disease is pituitary-dependent or adrenal-dependent. Adrenalectomy is the treatment of choice in cats with adrenal tumors.[34] In cats with PDH, bilateral adrenalectomy also has resulted in a successful outcome (**Fig. 7**).[34] The most successful drug for medical treatment of feline HAC is trilostane, but not all cats respond well to treatment.[43] The dose range of trilostane that has been reported to be effective in cats with PDH is 15 mg by mouth every 24 hours to 60 mg by mouth every 12 hours (**Fig. 8**).[37,43,47] Other drugs that have been used with limited success in cats with HAC include mitotane, metyrapone, and aminoglutethimide.[45,48–50] Other options in cats with PDH include hypophysectomy or radiation therapy.[28,29,41]

DIAGNOSTIC APPROACH TO INSULIN RESISTANCE IN CATS
Clinical Evaluation of Cats with Suspected Insulin Resistance

Assessment of cats with suspected insulin resistance requires performance of a BG curve, which should allow the clinician to rule out other causes of poor response to insulin (see **Box 1**). In cats receiving twice-daily insulin, a 12-hour BG curve is usually adequate. It is important to take into consideration the level of stress of the patient when interpreting the results of BG curves. It is also important to appreciate that BG curves show significant day-to-day variability.[51] Other measures such as clinical signs, results of urine and BG measurements at home, serum fructosamine concentrations, and changes in physical examination (especially body weight), should be taken into account when interpreting the results. Typically a BG curve in a cat with insulin resistance shows persistently high BG concentrations with no detectable nadir after insulin administration (see **Fig. 8**). Measurement of serum fructosamine is also useful in evaluation of cats with suspected insulin resistance. In cats with true insulin resistance, the fructosamine concentration is usually high, suggestive of poor glycemic control (**Table 2**). In cats with suspected insulin resistance in which fructosamine concentrations are consistent with good or moderate control, other causes of poor glycemic control should be considered. If the serum fructosamine concentration is low or in the reference range for a normal cat, insulin-induced hypoglycemia is the most likely cause of poor glycemic control.

The underlying cause of insulin resistance in cats usually can be identified by evaluation of historical findings, physical examination (including thorough oral

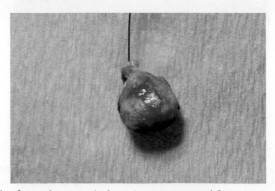

Fig. 7. Photograph of an adrenocortical carcinoma removed from a cat with signs of feminization caused by excess estradiol secretion from the tumor.

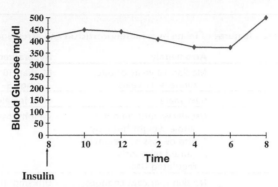

Fig. 8. Typical blood glucose curve in a cat with insulin resistance caused by acromegaly. Note the persistent increase in blood glucose and lack of a detectable nadir.

examination), and minimum database (CBC, biochemical profile, urinalysis, total T4) in addition to routine diagnostic tests such as urine culture, thoracic radiographs, abdominal ultrasound, and feline pancreatic enzyme assays. If this testing is unrewarding, the clinician should consider testing for concurrent endocrine disorders such as hyperadrenocorticism and acromegaly. The incidence of acromegaly in cats with severe insulin resistance appears to be higher than previously suspected, so in some cats it may be more appropriate to screen for acromegaly early in the work-up.[13,52] Clinical findings that would lead the clinician to be suspicious of acromegaly include absence of evidence of other underlying disease such as pancreatitis, heart disease, renal failure or hyperadrenocorticism, and a stable weight with no evidence of recurrent ketoacidosis (**Table 3**). Clinical signs that increase the index of suspicion for HAC include dermatologic signs, a pot-bellied appearance, persistent weight loss, and muscle atrophy. Adrenomegaly may be identified on abdominal ultrasound in cats with HAC, but because of the anabolic effects of IGF-1, cats with acromegaly also may have enlarged adrenal glands.

If no cause of insulin resistance can be identified in a cat with insulin resistance, strategies that may be useful for management of affected cats include an empiric change in diet or insulin formulation, attempts to control body weight in obese cats, and careful increases in insulin dose in cats with severe persistent insulin resistance. In cats with fluctuating insulin requirements, this approach may not be possible without risk of hypoglycemia. If no improvement in insulin sensitivity is observed, reevaluation is recommended in 2 to 3 months. In some cases, disease progression over time may make detection of underlying disease easier.

Table 2 Fructosamine concentrations in diabetic cats	
	Fructosamine Concentration (μmol/L)
Normal	142–450
Good control	<500
Fair control	500–614
Poor control	>614

Table 3
Comparison of clinical features of feline hyperadrenocorticism and acromegaly

	Acromegaly	Hyperadrenocorticism
Age	Median 10 years of age, range 4–17 years	Median 10 years of age, range 5–16 years
Sex	90% male	60% female
Body weight	Usually weight gain or stable weight but may also be loss of weight caused by poorly regulated DM	Weight loss is typical
Skin	No skin hair coat changes	Unkempt hair coat, alopecia, dermal and epidermal atrophy, cutaneous lacerations
Adrenal size	Normal to increased	Usually increased (either unilateral or bilateral)
Body size	Often larger cats affected, but cats may also be normal size	Body size is normal
Muscle mass	Normal muscle mass	Muscle atrophy common
Abdominal and thoracic organs	Renomegaly Hepatomegaly Cardiomegaly	Normal except for adrenals
Joints	Arthopathy	Normal
Predisposition to infection	Slightly predisposed because of DM	Marked increase in urinary tract infections, respiratory infections, and abscesses caused by both HAC and DM

SUMMARY

Most cats with true insulin resistance have underlying concurrent disease. The most common causes of insulin resistance are pancreatitis and bacterial infection. Acromegaly and HAC are important causes of insulin resistance in cats, and acromegaly may currently be underdiagnosed. Recent advances in definitive treatment of acromegaly and HAC may improve the quality of life and long-term survival of affected cats.

REFERENCES

1. Feldman EC, Nelson RW. Canine and feline endocrinology and reproduction. 3rd edition. Philadelphia: W.B. Saunders, Company; 2004.
2. Nelson RW, Lynn RC, Wagner-Mann CC, et al. Protamine zinc insulin for treatment of diabetes mellitus in cats. J Am Vet Med Assoc 2001;218:38–42.
3. Weaver KE, Rozanski EA, Mahoney OM, et al. Use of glargine and lente insulins in cats with diabetes mellitus. J Vet Intern Med 2006;20:234–8.
4. Martin GJ, Rand JS. Control of diabetes mellitus in cats with porcine insulin zinc suspension. Vet Rec 2007;161:88–94.
5. Bennett N, Greco DS, Peterson ME, et al. Comparisons of a low-carbohydrate low-fiber diet and a moderate-carbohydrate high-fiber diet in the management of feline diabetes mellitus. J Feline Med Surg 2006;8:73–84.

6. Rand JS, Kinnaird E, Bagliono A, et al. Acute stress hyperglycemia in cats is associated with struggling and increased concentrations of lactate and norepinephrine. J Vet Intern Med 2002;16:123–32.

7. Brushkiewicz KA, Nelson RW, Feldman EC, et al. Diabetic ketosis and ketoacidosis in cats: 42 cases (1980–1995). J Am Vet Med Assoc 1997;211:188–92.

8. Crenshaw KL, Peterson ME. Pretreatment clinical and laboratory evaluation of cats with diabetes mellitus: 104 cases (1992–1994). J Am Vet Med Assoc 1996;209:943–9.

9. Kraus MS, Calvert CA, Jacobs GJ, et al. Feline diabetes mellitus: a retrospective mortality study of 55 cats (1982–1994). J Am Anim Hosp Assoc 1997;33:107–11.

10. Little CJL, Gettinby G. Heart failure is common in diabetic cats: findings from a retrospective case-controlled study in first opinion practice. J Small Anim Pract 2008;49:17–25.

11. Goosens MMC, Nelson RW, Feldman EC, et al. Response to insulin treatment and survival in 104 cats with diabetes mellitus (1985–1995). J Vet Intern Med 1998;12:1–6.

12. Bailiff NL, Nelson RW, Feldman EC, et al. Frequency and risk factors for urinary tract infection in cats with diabetes mellitus. J Vet Intern Med 2006;20:850–5.

13. Slingerland LI, Voorhout G, Rijnberk A, et al. Growth hormone excess and the effect of octreotide in cats with diabetes mellitus. Domest Anim Endocrinol 2008;35:352–61.

14. Niessen SJ, Petrie G, Gaudiano F, et al. Feline acromegaly: an underdiagnosed endocrinopathy? J Vet Intern Med 2007;21:899–905.

15. Berg RI, Nelson RW, Feldman EC, et al. Serum insulin-like growth factor-I concentration in cats with diabetes mellitus and acromegaly. J Vet Intern Med 2007;21:892–8.

16. Slingerland LI, Fazilova VV, Plantinga EA, et al. Indoor confinement and physical inactivity rather than the proportion of dry food are risk factors in the development of feline type 2 diabetes mellitus. Vet J 2009;179:247–53.

17. Hoenig M, Thoaseth K, Brandao J, et al. Assessment and mathematical modeling of glucose turnover and insulin sensitivity in lean and obese cats. Domest Anim Endocrinol 2006;31:373–89.

18. Forman MA, Marks SL, De Cock HEV, et al. Evaluation of serum feline pancreatic lipase immunoreactivity and helical computed tomography versus conventional testing for the diagnosis of feline pancreatitis. J Vet Intern Med 2004;18:807–15.

19. Hoenig M, Ferguson DC. Impairment of glucose tolerance in hyperthyroid cats. J Endocrinol 1989;121:249–51.

20. Hoenig M. Glucose tolerance and insulin secretion in spontaneously hyperthyroid cats. Res Vet Sci 1992;53:338–41.

21. Peterson ME, Melián C, Nichols R. Measurement of serum concentrations of free thyroxine, total thyroxine, and total triiodothyronine in cats with hyperthyroidism and cats with nonthyroidal disease. J Am Vet Med Assoc 2001;218:529–36.

22. Hurty CA, Flatland B. Feline acromegaly: a review of the syndrome. J Am Anim Hosp Assoc 2005;41:292–7.

23. Peterson ME, Taylor RS, Greco DS, et al. Acromegaly in 14 cats. J Vet Intern Med 1000;4:102 201.

24. Peterson ME. Acromegaly in cats: are we only diagnosing the tip of the iceberg? J Vet Intern Med 2007;21:889–91.

25. Starkey SR, Tan K, Church DB. Investigation of serum IGF-1 levels amongst diabetic and nondiabetic cats. J Feline Med Surg 2004;6:149–55.

26. Niessen SJM, Khalid M, Petrie G, et al. Validation and application of a radioimmunoassay for ovine growth hormone in the diagnosis of acromegaly in cats. Vet Rec 2007;160:902–7.
27. Reusch CE, Kley S, Casella M. Measurement of growth hormone and insulin-like growth factor 1 in cats with diabetes mellitus. Vet Rec 2006;158:195–200.
28. Kaser-Hotz B, Rohrer CR, Stankeova S, et al. Radiotherapy of pituitary tumors in five cats. J Small Anim Pract 2002;43:303–7.
29. Mayer MN, Greco DS, LaRue SM. Outcomes of pituitary irradiation in cats. J Vet Intern Med 2006;20:1151–4.
30. Dunning MD, Lowrie CS, Bexfield NH, et al. Exogenous insulin treatment after hypofractionated radiotherapy in cats with diabetes mellitus and acromegaly. J Vet Intern Med 2009;23:243–9.
31. Goosens MM, Feldman EC, Nelson RW, et al. Cobalt 60 irradiation of pituitary gland tumors in three cats with acromegaly. J Am Vet Med Assoc 1998;213: 374–6.
32. Blois SL, Holmberg D. Cryohypophysectomy used in the treatment of a case of feline acromegaly. J Small Anim Pract 2008;49:596–600.
33. Nelson RW, Feldman EC, Smith MC. Hyperadrenocorticism in cats: seven cases (1978–1987). J Am Vet Med Assoc 1988;193(2):245–50.
34. Duesberg CA, Nelson RW, Feldman EC, et al. Adrenalectomy for treatment of hyperadrenocorticism in cats: 10 cases (1988–1992). J Am Vet Med Assoc 1995; 207:1066–70.
35. Watson PJ, Herrtage ME. Hyperadrenocorticism in six cats. J Small Anim Pract 1998;39:175–84.
36. DeClue AE, Breshears LA, Pardo ID, et al. Hyperaldosteronism and hyperprogesteronemia in a cat with an adrenal cortical carcinoma. J Vet Intern Med 2005;19: 355–8.
37. Boag AK, Neiger R, Church DB. Trilostane treatment of bilateral adrenal enlargement and excessive sex steroid hormone production in a cat. J Small Anim Pract 2004;45:263–6.
38. De Lange MS, Galac S, Trip MRJ, et al. High urinary corticoid: creatinine ratios in cats with hyperthyroidism. J Vet Intern Med 2004;18:152–5.
39. Henry CJ, Clark TP, Young DW, et al. Urine cortisol: creatinine ratio in healthy and sick cats. J Vet Intern Med 1996;10:123–6.
40. Goosens MMC, Meyer HP, Voorhout G, et al. Urinary excretion of glucocorticoids in the diagnosis of hyperadrenocorticism in cats. Domest Anim Endocrinol 1995; 12:355–62.
41. Meij BP, Voorhout G, Van Den Ingh TS, et al. Transsphenoidal hypophysectomy for treatment of pituitary dependent hyperadrenocorticism in 7 cats. Vet Surg 2001;30:72–86.
42. Peterson ME, Kemppainen RJ. Comparison of intravenous and intramuscular routes of administering cosyntropin for corticotropin stimulation testing in cats. Am J Vet Res 1992;53:1392–5.
43. Neiger RN, Witt AL, Noble A, et al. Trilostane therapy for treatment of pituitary-dependent hyperadrenocorticism in 5 cats. J Vet Intern Med 2004;18: 160–4.
44. Boord M, Griffin C. Progesterone secreting adrenal mass in a cat with clinical signs of hyperadrenocorticism. J Am Vet Med Assoc 1999;214:666–9.
45. Rossmeisl JH, Scott-Moncrieff JC, Siems J, et al. Hyperadrencorticism and hyperprogesteronemia in a cat with an adrenocortical adenocarcinoma. J Am Anim Hosp Assoc 2000;36:512–7.

46. Zimmer C, Hörauf A, Reusch C. Ultrasonographic examination of the adrenal gland and evaluation of the hypophyseal-adrenal axis in 20 cats. J Small Anim Pract 2000;41:156–60.
47. Skelly BJ, Petrus D, Nicholls PK. Use of trilostane for the treatment of pituitary-dependent hyperadrenocorticism in a cat. J Small Anim Pract 2003;44:269–72.
48. Moore LE, Biller DS, Olsen DE. Hyperadrenocorticism treated with metyrapone followed by bilateral adrenalectomy in a cat. J Am Vet Med Assoc 2000;217: 691–4.
49. Schwedes CS. Mitotane (op'-DDD) treatment in a cat with hyperadrenocorticism. J Small Anim Pract 1997;38:520–4.
50. Daley CA, Zerbe CA, Schick RO, et al. Use of metyrapone to treat pituitary-dependent hyperadrenocorticism in a cat with large cutaneous wounds. J Am Vet Med Assoc 1993;202:956–60.
51. Alt N, Kley S, Haessig M, et al. Day to day variability of blood glucose concentration curves generated at home in cats with diabetes mellitus. J Am Vet Med Assoc 2007;230:1011–7.
52. Elliott DA, Feldman EC, Koblik PD, et al. Prevalence of pituitary tumors among diabetic cats with insulin resistance. J Am Vet Med Assoc 2000;216:1765–8.

56. Zeugswetter F, Pagitz M. Ketone measurements using dipstick methodology in cats with diabetes mellitus. J Am Vet Med Assoc 2009;45:4–8.

57. Tschuor F, Zini E, Schellenberg S, et al. Evaluation of four portable blood glucose meters for measurement of blood glucose concentrations in cats. J Am Vet Med Assoc 2009;235:1438–42.

58. Wess G, Reusch C. Assessment of five portable blood glucose meters for use in cats. Am J Vet Res 2000;61:1587–92.

59. Sennello KA, Schulman RL, Prosek R, et al. Systolic blood pressure in cats with diabetes mellitus. J Am Vet Med Assoc 2003;223:198–201.

60. Bloom CA, Rand JS. Diabetes and the kidney in human and veterinary medicine. Vet Clin North Am Small Anim Pract 2013;43:351–65.

61. Zini E, Hafner M, Osto M, et al. Predictors of clinical remission in cats with diabetes mellitus. J Vet Intern Med 2010;24:1314–21.

62. Reusch CE, Liehs MR, Hoyer M, et al. Fructosamine. A new parameter for diagnosis and metabolic control in diabetic dogs and cats. J Vet Intern Med 1993;7:177–82.

Recent Advances in the Diagnosis of Cushing's Syndrome in Dogs

Hans S. Kooistra, DVM, PhD*, Sara Galac, DVM

KEYWORDS

- Hypercortisolism • Pituitary-adrenocortical axis
- Urinary corticoids • Adrenocorticotropic hormone
- Diagnostic imaging

Hypercortisolism is a common condition in dogs and can be defined as the physical and biochemical changes that result from prolonged exposure to inappropriately high plasma concentrations of (free) cortisol, whatever its' cause. This disorder is often called Cushing's syndrome, after Harvey Cushing, the neurosurgeon who first described the human syndrome in 1932.

Cushing's syndrome is sometimes iatrogenic, in most cases due to administration of glucocorticoids for the treatment of a variety of allergic, autoimmune, inflammatory, or neoplastic diseases. The development of clinical signs of glucocorticoid excess depends on the severity and duration of the exposure. The effects also vary among animals owing to interindividual differences in cortisol sensitivity. Corticosteroid administration causes prompt and sustained suppression of the hypothalamic-pituitary-adrenocortical axis. Depending on the dose and the intrinsic glucocorticoid activity of the corticosteroid, the schedule and duration of its administration, and the preparation or formulation, this suppression may exist for weeks or months after cessation of the corticosteroid administration.

This article focuses on the diagnosis of spontaneous hypercortisolism. In 80% to 85% of the spontaneous cases, hypercortisolism is adrenocorticotropic hormone (ACTH)-dependent, usually arising from hypersecretion of ACTH by a pituitary corticotroph adenoma. Ectopic ACTH-secretion syndrome is rare in dogs.[1] The remaining 15% to 20% of cases of spontaneous hypercortisolism are ACTH-independent and result from autonomous hypersecretion of glucocorticoids by an adrenocortical adenoma or adenocarcinoma. In addition to an adrenocortical tumor, ACTH-independent hypercortisolism can be caused by bilateral (macro)nodular adrenocortical

Department of Clinical Sciences of Companion Animals, Faculty of Veterinary Medicine, Utrecht University, Yalelaan 108, 3584 CM Utrecht, The Netherlands
* Corresponding author.
E-mail address: H.S.Kooistra@uu.nl (H.S. Kooistra).

Vet Clin Small Anim 40 (2010) 259–267
doi:10.1016/j.cvsm.2009.10.002
0195-5616/10/$ – see front matter © 2010 Elsevier Inc. All rights reserved.

vetsmall.theclinics.com

hyperplasia because of aberrant adrenal expression of either ectopic or overactive eutopic hormone receptors.[2–4]

CLINICAL MANIFESTATIONS OF HYPERCORTISOLISM

All endocrine tests used for the diagnosis of endogenous hypercortisolism entail measurement of cortisol in plasma or urine (or saliva). Regardless of which test is used, a high degree of clinical suspicion is mandatory to avoid false-positive test results. Positive test results in patients that have developed several clinical signs of Cushing's syndrome over a relatively short period of time are more likely to be diagnostic than positive test results obtained in patients with more unusual presentations. Obviously, presentations that are more unusual require more confirmatory tests than a dog with a typical history and clear-cut physical and biochemical changes. Notably, several dogs with Cushing's syndrome do not present the full-blown picture originally described in textbooks. Instead, they often have milder hypercortisolism with less pronounced symptomatology. Thus, making a diagnosis requires considerable clinical insight.

Spontaneous hypercortisolism is a disease of middle-aged and older dogs, although, very rarely, it may occur as early as 1 year of age. There is no gender predilection. It occurs in all dog breeds, with a slight predilection for small breeds such as dachshunds and miniature poodles. The incidence is much higher in dogs than in humans and cats and has been reported to be 1 to 2 cases per 1000 dogs per year.[5]

Many of the clinical signs can be related to the biochemical effects of glucocorticoids, namely increased gluconeogenesis and lipogenesis at the expense of protein (**Fig. 1**). In dogs, the cardinal physical features are centripetal obesity and atrophy of muscles and skin (**Fig. 2**). Polyuria and polyphagia are also dominating features. The polyuria is known to be due to impaired osmoregulation of vasopressin release and interference of the glucocorticoid excess with the action of vasopressin in the

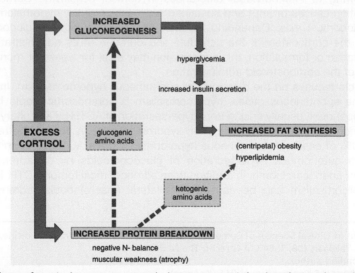

Fig. 1. Effects of cortisol excess. Increased gluconeogenesis leads to hyperglycemia, which is controlled initially by increased insulin secretion. This causes increased lipogenesis. Thus, the result of glucocorticoid excess is the catabolism of peripheral tissues such as muscle and skin to deliver the substrate for increased gluconeogenesis and lipogenesis.

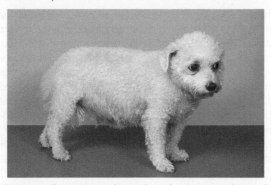

Fig. 2. A 9-year-old dog with pituitary-dependent hypercortisolism. The hypercortisolism resulted in a thin hair coat and an enlarged abdomen. Furthermore, the dog had polyuria and polyphagia.

kidney. Abdominal palpation may reveal hepatomegaly. For a complete overview of the clinical signs related to hypercortisolism the reader is referred to the work of Galac and colleagues.[6]

Increased plasma alkaline phosphatase (AP) activity is a frequent finding in dogs with hypercortisolism. This is mainly because of the induction of an isoenzyme having greater stability at 65°C than other AP-isoenzymes and, therefore, easily measured by a routine laboratory procedure.[7] In about 50% of dogs with hypercortisolism plasma thyroxine (T$_4$) is decreased as a consequence of altered transport, distribution, and metabolism of T$_4$, rather than due to hyposecretion. For a complete overview of the changes in routine laboratory data related to hypercortisolism the reader is again referred to the work of Galac and colleagues.[6]

Diagnostic imaging may help to complete the picture of the physical and biochemical changes associated with glucocorticoid excess. Although hepatomegaly and a distended urinary bladder may be seen, abdominal radiography is of little use in the diagnostic work-up of a dog suspected of having hypercortisolism. Thoracic radiographs may show bronchial and interstitial mineralization.[8] Dystrophic calcification in the skin and subcutis may also be seen in the areas of predilection for calcinosis cutis. Ultrasonography, CT, and MRI are the imaging techniques used most frequently, especially in characterization of the source of the hormone excess.

DIAGNOSIS OF HYPERCORTISOLISM

The endocrine diagnosis of hypercortisolism depends on the demonstration of two principal characteristics of all forms of the condition: (1) increased production of cortisol and (2) decreased sensitivity to glucocorticoid feedback. Measurement of a single plasma cortisol concentration has little diagnostic value because the pulsatile secretion of ACTH results in variable plasma cortisol concentrations that may at times be within the reference range. There are two ways to overcome this problem: (1) to test the integrity of the feedback system, and (2) to measure urinary corticoid excretion.

In the first approach, the sensitivity of the pituitary-adrenocortical system to suppression is tested by administering a synthetic glucocorticoid in a dose that discriminates between healthy dogs and dogs with hypercortisolism. A potent glucocorticoid such as dexamethasone is used so that the dose will be too small to contribute significantly to the laboratory measurement. In this so-called dexamethasone screening test or low-dose dexamethasone suppression test (LDDST),

0.01 mg dexamethasone per kg body weight is administered intravenously (IV). Blood for cortisol measurement is collected before, and 4 hours and 8 hours after dexamethasone administration. The finding of a plasma cortisol concentration exceeding 40 nmol/L at 8 hours after dexamethasone administration, in dogs with physical and biochemical changes pointing to hypercortisolism, confirms hypercortisolism with a predictive value of a positive test result of 0.92 (and a predictive value of a negative test result of 0.59).[9] The measurements at 0 hour and 4 hours are not needed for the diagnosis per se but may be useful in the differential diagnosis. If the plasma cortisol concentration at either 4 hours or 8 hours is at least 50% lower than the 0-hour value, the hypercortisolism is pituitary-dependent. The iv-LDDST can have a false-positive result because of stress, for example because of the hospital visit and blood collection.[10]

This IV-LDDST is increasingly replaced by the measurement of urinary corticoids. Because urine is stored and mixed in the bladder for several hours, an integrated reflection of corticoid production is obtained, thereby adjusting for fluctuations in plasma concentrations. The urinary corticoids (largely cortisol) are related to the creatinine concentration in the urine, resulting in the urinary corticoid to creatinine ratio (UCCR). This test requires little time (from the veterinarian and the owner), is not invasive (no blood collection), and has a high diagnostic accuracy. In addition, the test procedure has the advantage of combining a test for basal adrenocortical function and a dynamic test for differential diagnosis (see below). To avoid the influence of stress, the urine for the UCCR determination has to be collected at home, at least 1 day after the visit of the veterinary clinic. Nonadrenal disease may also result in endogenous stress and elevated cortisol secretion and, therefore, high UCCRs in dogs that do not have a high degree of clinical suspicion should be interpreted with care. The owner collects a morning urine sample on 2 consecutive days and the UCCRs in these two samples are averaged. In our laboratory, the basal UCCR in healthy pet dogs varies from 0.3 to 8.3×10^{-6}.[11] In dogs with physical and biochemical changes pointing to hypercortisolism the predictive value of a positive test result is 0.88 and that of a negative test result is 0.98.[9] In some dogs there is considerable day-to-day variation in the UCCR, which in mild forms of hypercortisolism occasionally leads to UCCRs just within the reference range, whereas collections on other days might have revealed one or two elevated UCCRs. The uncertainty can be resolved by measuring the UCCR in urine samples collected on 10 consecutive days.

In dogs in which results of the UCCR or the IV-LDDST have been inconclusive or negative but in which there is still suspicion of hypercortisolism, an oral LDDST may be performed. The owner collects urine at 8.00 hours (at home) for measurement of the UCCR. After collection of the urine sample, the owner administers 0.01 mg dexamethasone per kg body weight orally. The dog is walked at 12.00 hours and 14.00 hours to empty its bladder and the second urine sample is collected at 16.00 hours for measurement of UCCR. In seven healthy pet dogs, the UCCR at 16.00 hours was less than 1.0×10^{-6}.[12] In dogs with mild pituitary-dependent hypercortisolism, the UCCR following dexamethasone was greater than 1.0×10^{-6}.[13]

Another popular test to screen for hypercortisolism is the ACTH stimulation test. The main indication for the ACTH stimulation test is to test the adrenocortical reserve capacity; that is, to diagnose primary or secondary adrenocortical insufficiency. Thus, the ACTH stimulation test can be used very well to diagnose iatrogenic hypercorticism. In cases of spontaneous hypercortisolism, ACTH stimulation may result in an exaggerated adrenal response; that is, a higher plasma cortisol concentration than in healthy dogs. About 85% of dogs with pituitary-dependent hypercortisolism have exaggerated cortisol responses to ACTH, while only about 55% of dogs with hypercortisolism due to adrenocortical tumor have such a result.[14] The main advantages of the ACTH stimulation test are its simplicity and the short duration of the test. However, the diagnostic accuracy for hypercortisolism of this test is less than that of the UCCR and the LDDST. Therefore, this test is no longer recommended in the diagnostic approach of dogs with hypercortisolism.[15]

When hypercortisolism has been confirmed, it is necessary to distinguish between the different forms of the disease.

PITUITARY-DEPENDENT HYPERCORTISOLISM

In most cases, ACTH-dependent hypercortisolism arises from hypersecretion of ACTH by a pituitary corticotroph adenoma. The ACTH excess may originate in both the anterior lobe and the pars intermedia of the pituitary gland. In about 75% to 80% of cases, there is an adenoma in the anterior lobe.[16,17] Despite decreased sensitivity to glucocorticoid feedback, the hallmark of Cushing's syndrome, (a high dose of) dexamethasone can suppress ACTH secretion in most dogs with pituitary-dependent hypercortisolism (PDH) due to a corticotroph adenoma in the anterior lobe.

In about one-fourth to one-fifth of cases there is a corticotroph adenoma in the pars intermedia.[16,17] This is of clinical interest, not only because the pars intermedia tumors tend to be larger than anterior lobe tumors,[16] but also because of the specific hypothalamic control of hormone synthesis in the pars intermedia. The pars intermedia is under direct neural control, principally tonic dopaminergic inhibition,[18] which suppresses the expression of glucocorticoid receptors. This explains why PDH of pars intermedia origin is resistant to suppression by dexamethasone. In other forms of spontaneous hypercortisolism, the hypersecretion of cortisol is not dependent on pituitary ACTH and is therefore also not influenced by the administration of dexamethasone.

The impaired sensitivity to glucocorticoid feedback in PDH due to an anterior lobe tumor can be demonstrated by performing a high-dose dexamethasone suppression test (HDDST). Two procedures are used, one employing plasma cortisol and the other employing the UCCR. In both, a decrease of more than 50% from baseline values confirms PDH.[19] For the IV-HDDST, blood for measurement of plasma cortisol concentrations is collected immediately before and 3 to 4 hours after intravenous administration of 0.1 mg dexamethasone per kg body weight. When UCCRs are used, the owner has to administer three oral doses of dexamethasone (0.1 mg per kg body weight) at 8-hour intervals after collection of the second basal urine sample (see above). As mentioned earlier, the urine samples should be collected by the owner at home under conditions free of stress.[11]

When there is less than 50% suppression, the hypercortisolism may still be pituitary-dependent, due to either a pars intermedia tumor or a resistant anterior lobe tumor. Further differentiation requires measurements of plasma ACTH concentrations. In animals with PDH, plasma ACTH concentrations are not completely suppressed despite high plasma cortisol concentrations.[20]

When PDH has been proven, the pituitary gland can be detected by CT or MRI. Pituitary imaging is necessary if either hypophysectomy or pituitary irradiation is to be used for treatment,[21] but also provides information with regard to the prognosis. Dynamic contrast enhanced CT facilitates contrast enhancement of the neurohypophysis and the adenohypophysis. Absence of the pituitary flush indicates atrophy of the neurohypophysis due to compression by a pituitary tumor. Displacement or distortion of the pituitary flush in the early phase of dynamic CT can be used to identify and localize microadenomas originating from the anterior lobe or pars intermedia in dogs.[22]

HYPERCORTISOLISM DUE TO AN ADRENOCORTICAL TUMOR

Hypersecretion of cortisol by an adrenocortical tumor (AT) cannot be suppressed by administration of dexamethasone. As indicated by either plasma cortisol concentration or the UCCR, resistance to suppression by a high dose of dexamethasone is, with similar probability, due to AT or dexamethasone-resistant PDH.[19] In some dogs with a cortisol-secreting AT, dexamethasone causes a paradoxic rise in both the UCCR and plasma cortisol.[19] Hypercortisolism due to AT can be differentiated from nonsuppressible forms of PDH by measuring the plasma ACTH concentration. In addition, an AT is often readily detected by ultrasonography. Hence, it is common practice in cases of nonsuppressible hypercortisolism to measure the plasma ACTH concentration and to perform ultrasonography of the adrenal glands. If an AT is found, ACTH measurement is still useful. Plasma ACTH concentrations should be low. If not, further studies are warranted to determine if PDH is also present.[23]

A recent study showed that intravenous administration of 4 μg desmopressin (DDAVP) did not increase plasma cortisol concentration in seven dogs with AT, whereas 75% of 46 dogs with PDH had increases in plasma cortisol concentrations of more than 10% compared with baseline concentrations.[24] The results of this study suggest that a desmopressin stimulation test may be a useful tool in differentiating PDH from AT, but additional dogs with AT must be tested before this test can be recommended in clinical practice.

The preferred procedures for imaging of the adrenal glands are MRI and CT. Ultrasonography is less expensive, requires less time and usually no anesthesia, and so it is often used first even though it is more difficult to perform and to interpret than CT or MRI. Ultrasonography provides a good estimate of the size of the tumor and may reveal information about its expansion.[25,26] Because it is sometimes difficult to distinguish between (macro)nodular hyperplasia and AT by ultrasonography, CT or MRI may be needed. Most ATs are unilateral solitary lesions, the two glands being affected about equally, but bilateral tumors occur in approximately 10% of cases.[26–28]

When an AT has been confirmed, the possibility of distant metastases should be considered. During abdominal ultrasonography, the liver should be examined for metastases. If possible metastases are found, ultrasound-guided biopsy can be performed. Thoracic radiography or a CT scan of the thorax should be performed to exclude metastases in the lungs.

HYPERCORTISOLISM DUE TO ECTOPIC ACTH SECRETION

Ectopic ACTH hypersecretion has been documented in an 8-year-old German shepherd dog.[1] The UCCRs and plasma ACTH concentrations were very high and not suppressible with dexamethasone. These findings were initially interpreted as being consistent with PDH. However, histologic examination of the tissue removed by transsphenoidal hypophysectomy did not confirm the presence of an adenoma. Within 2 weeks after hypophysectomy the clinical manifestations were exacerbated and both the UCCR and plasma ACTH concentration were further increased. CT of the abdomen revealed a tumor in the region of the pancreas. Laparotomy revealed a 5-mm nodule in the pancreas, a 3-cm metastasis in an adjacent lymph node, and metastases in the liver. Partial pancreatectomy and excision of the lymph node were performed, and a neuroendocrine tumor with metastasis in the lymph node was diagnosed by histopathology. Based on this report, ectopic ACTH secretion should be considered in cases of severe hypercortisolism in which plasma ACTH concentrations are very high and are not suppressible with high doses of dexamethasone, and in which diagnostic imaging does not reveal a pituitary tumor. In patients with PDH, intravenous administration of 1 μg corticotropin-releasing hormone (CRH) per kg body weight results in a significant increase in plasma concentrations of ACTH and cortisol; but in patients with ectopic ACTH secretion CRH does not increase these plasma hormone concentrations.[1] The neuroendocrine tumor causing the ectopic ACTH syndrome may be detected by a whole-body scan, but in human patients with ectopic ACTH syndrome the tumors are frequently small and often not found. Based on reports of individual cases in which ectopic ACTH secretion may have caused hypercortisolism, the condition may not be extremely rare in dogs.[29,30]

HYPERCORTISOLISM DUE TO ECTOPIC OR HYPERACTIVE EUTOPIC ADRENOCORTICAL RECEPTORS

In addition to autonomous cortisol secretion by an AT, ACTH-independent hypercortisolism can also be caused by aberrant adrenal expression of either ectopic or over-expressed eutopic hormone receptors.[2,3] Most of these hormone receptors belong to the superfamily of G protein-coupled receptors.[31] In humans, various adrenocortical membrane-bound receptors functionally coupled to steroidogenesis have been reported, including glucose-dependent insulinotropic polypeptide (GIP), catecholamine, vasopressin, serotonin, and luteinizing hormone receptors.

In a recently published case report of a dog with food-dependent hypercortisolism, the ACTH-independent hypercortisolism was most likely due to aberrant adrenocortical expression of GIP receptors.[4] The hormone GIP is secreted in the gastrointestinal tract in response to a meal and normally serves to enhance postprandial insulin secretion. In human patients with aberrant adrenocortical expression of GIP receptors, a meal not only results in augmented insulin secretion but also in increased steroidogenesis. The dog described in the case report had clinical manifestations of hypercortisolism and slightly elevated UCCRs. Basal and CRH-stimulated plasma ACTH concentrations were low, but diagnostic imaging did not reveal an adrenocortical tumor. Ingestion of a meal resulted in significant increases in plasma cortisol concentration and UCCR. Consistent with the diagnostic criteria for food-dependent hypercortisolism in humans,[2,32] IV administration of 3 μg octreotide per kg body weight completely prevented the meal-induced hypercortisolemia. The dog had a good clinical response to medical treatment with trilostane, administered shortly before the main meal.

Thus, a distinct increase in UCCR and plasma cortisol concentration after ingestion of a meal,[4] low or undetectable plasma ACTH concentrations, and prevention of a meal-induced rise in plasma cortisol concentration by octreotide administration strongly suggest food-dependent hypercortisolism.

SUMMARY

The recognition of new causes of hypercortisolism, such as ectopic ACTH secretion and food-dependent hypercortisolism, and changes in technology, such as advances in imaging procedures, have reshaped the diagnostic scenario. An array of tests is available for the diagnosis of Cushing's syndrome, but once the diagnosis of hypercortisolism is made considerable expertise is still required to determine its cause, to allow selection of the best treatment, and to avoid misdiagnosis.

REFERENCES

1. Galac S, Kooistra HS, Voorhout G, et al. Hyperadrenocorticism in a dog due to ectopic secretion of adrenocorticotropic hormone. Domest Anim Endocrinol 2005;28:338–48.

2. Lacroix A, N'Diaye N, Tremblay J, et al. Ectopic and abnormal hormone receptors in adrenal Cushing's syndrome. Endocr Rev 2001;22:75–110.
3. Christopoulos S, Bordeau I, Lacroix A. Clinical and subclinical ACTH-independent macronodular hyperplasia and aberrant hormone receptors. Horm Res 2005;64:119–31.
4. Galac S, Kars VJ, Voorhout G, et al. ACTH-independent hyperadrenocorticism due to food-dependent hypercortisolemia in a dog: a case report. Vet J 2008; 177:141–3.
5. Willeberg P, Priester WA. Epidemiological aspects of clinical hyperadrenocorticism in dogs (canine Cushing's syndrome). J Am Anim Hosp Assoc 1982;18: 717–24.
6. Galac S, Reusch CE, Kooistra HS, et al. Adrenals. In: Rijnberk A, Kooistra HS, editors. Clinical endocrinology of dogs and cats. 2nd edition. Hannover (Germany): Schlütersche; 2010, in press.
7. Teske E, Rothuizen J, de Bruijne JJ, et al. Corticosteroid-induced alkaline phosphatase isoenzyme in the diagnosis of canine hypercorticism. Vet Rec 1989;125: 12–4.
8. Berry CR, Hawkins EC, Hurley KJ, et al. Frequency of pulmonary mineralization and hypoxemia in 21 dogs with pituitary-dependent hyperadrenocorticism. J Vet Intern Med 2000;14:151–6.
9. Rijnberk A, van Wees A, Mol JA. Assessment of two tests for the diagnosis of canine hyperadrenocorticism. Vet Rec 1988;122:178–80.
10. Chastain CB, Franklin RT, Ganjam VK, et al. Evaluation of the hypothalamic pituitary-adrenal axis in clinically stressed dogs. J Am Anim Hosp Assoc 1986;22: 435–42.
11. Van Vonderen IK, Kooistra HS, Rijnberk A. Intra- and interindividual variation in urine osmolality and urine specific gravity in healthy pet dogs of various ages. J Vet Intern Med 1997;11:30–5.
12. Vaessen MM, Kooistra HS, Mol JA, et al. Urinary corticoid:creatinine ratios in healthy pet dogs after oral low-dose dexamethasone suppression tests. Vet Rec 2004;155:518–21.
13. Cerundolo R, Lloyd DH, Vaessen MM, et al. Alopecia in pomeranians and miniature poodles in association with high urinary corticoid:creatinine ratios and resistance to glucocorticoid feedback. Vet Rec 2007;160:393–7.
14. Peterson ME, Gilbertson SR, Drucker WD. Plasma cortisol response to exogenous ACTH in 22 dogs with hyperadrenocorticism caused by adrenocortical neoplasia. J Am Vet Med Assoc 1982;180:542–4.
15. Feldman EC. Treatment of hyperadrenocorticism in dogs. In: Proceedings ACVIM Forum; 2005. p. 672–5.
16. Peterson ME, Krieger DT, Drucker WD, et al. Immunocytochemical study of the hypophysis of 25 dogs with pituitary-dependent hyperadrenocorticism. Acta Endocrinol 1982;101:15–24.
17. Peterson ME, Orth DN, Halmi NS, et al. Plasma immunoreactive proopiomelanocortin peptides and cortisol in normal dogs and dogs with Addison's disease and Cushing's syndrome: basal concentrations. Endocrinology 1986;119:720–30.
18. Kemppainen RJ, Sartin JL. Differential regulation of peptide release by the canine pars distalis and pars intermedia. Front Horm Res 1987;17:18–27.
19. Galac S, Kooistra HS, Teske E, et al. Urinary corticoid/creatinine ratios in the differentiation between pituitary-dependent hyperadrenocorticism and hyperadrenocorticism due to adrenocortical tumour in the dog. Vet Q 1997;19: 17–20.

20. Gould SM, Baines EA, Mannion PA, et al. Use of endogenous ACTH concentration and adrenal ultrasonography to distinguish the cause of canine hyperadrenocorticism. J Small Anim Pract 2001;42:113–21.
21. Van der Vlugt-Meijer RH, Voorhout G, Meij BP. Imaging of the pituitary gland in dogs with pituitary-dependent hyperadrenocorticism. Mol Cell Endocrinol 2002; 197:81–7.
22. Van der Vlugt-Meijer RH, Meij BP, van den Ingh TS, et al. Dynamic computed tomography of the pituitary gland in dogs with pituitary-dependent hyperadrenocorticism. J Vet Intern Med 2003;17:773–80.
23. Greco DS, Peterson ME, Davidson AP, et al. Concurrent pituitary and adrenal tumors in dogs with hyperadrenocorticism: 17 cases (1978–1995). J Am Vet Med Assoc 1999;214:1349–53.
24. Zeugswetter F, Hoyer MT, Pagitz M, et al. The desmopressin stimulation test in dogs with Cushing's syndrome. Domest Anim Endocrinol 2008;34:254–60.
25. Voorhout G, Rijnberk A, Sjollema BE, et al. Nephrotomography and ultrasonography for the localization of hyperfunctioning adrenocortical tumors in dogs. Am J Vet Res 1990;51:1280–5.
26. Hoerauf A, Reusch CE. Ultrasonographic characteristics of both adrenal glands in 15 dogs with functional adrenocortical tumors. J Am Anim Hosp Assoc 1999; 35:193–9.
27. Ford SL, Feldman EC, Nelson RW. Hyperadrenocorticism caused by bilateral adrenocortical neoplasia in dogs: four cases (1983–1988). J Am Vet Med Assoc 1993;202:789–92.
28. Van Sluijs FJ, Sjollema BE, Voorhout G, et al. Results of adrenalectomy in 36 dogs with hyperadrenocorticism caused by adrenocortical tumour. Vet Q 1995;17: 113–6.
29. Churcher RK. Hepatic carcinoid, hypercortisolism and hypokalaemia in a dog. Aust Vet J 1999;77:641–5.
30. Burgener IA, Gerold A, Tomek A, et al. Empty sella syndrome, hyperadrenocorticism and megaoesophagus in a dachshund. J Small Anim Pract 2007;48:584–7.
31. Schorr I, Ney RL. Abnormal hormone responses of an adrenocortical cancer adenyl cyclase. J Clin Invest 1971;50:1295–300.
32. Croughs RJ, Zellissen PM, van Vroonhoven TJ, et al. GIP-dependent adrenal Cushing's syndrome with incomplete suppression of ACTH. J Clin Endocrinol Metab 2000;52:235–40.

Trilostane in Dogs

Ian K. Ramsey, BVSc, PhD

KEYWORDS

• Hyperadrenocorticism • Treatment • Adrenal
• Steroid synthesis inhibitor

Trilostane (4,5-epoxy-17-hydroxy-3-oxoandrostane-2-carbonitrile) is a synthetic steroid whose ability to reduce adrenocorticotropic hormone (ACTH) stimulation of adrenal corticoids was first described 40 years ago.[1] Further studies demonstrated that it was orally active and that its mode of action was as a competitive inhibitor of steroid synthesis.[2] The use of trilostane was investigated in various human conditions, including hyperadrenocorticism (HAC), hyperaldosteronism, and breast cancer.[3–7] Although it did appear to have some effect on some cases of human HAC, it was not as effective as other available treatments and, in a recent consensus statement, is no longer considered as a treatment option.[8] It is, however, still used in the treatment of human breast cancer.[9]

The first report of the use of trilostane in canine HAC was by Hurley and colleagues[10] who successfully treated a series of 15 dogs, including 2 with adrenal-dependent disease. In the following decade, many other abstracts and articles followed. Trilostane was first authorized in the United Kingdom in 2005 for the treatment of canine HAC but has since been authorized in many other countries, most recently in the United States. Formulations for human use and imported veterinary formulations are often used in those countries where it is not currently authorized for veterinary use.

The information contained within this article is intended for an international audience, and some information (eg, doses) may be at variance with national recommendations. Veterinarians should consult their national regulatory authorities or local commercial representatives if they are unsure as to their local rules and guidelines.

MODE OF ACTION

Trilostane is a competitive inhibitor of the 3β-hydroxysteroid dehydrogenase/isomerase system (3β-HSD), an essential enzyme system for the synthesis of several steroids, including cortisol and aldosterone.[2] This enzyme catalyzes the conversion of the 3β-hydroxysteroids (pregnenolone, 17-hydroxypregnenolone, and dehydroepiandrosterone [DHEA]) to the 3-ketosteroids (progesterone,

Faculty of Veterinary Medicine, University of Glasgow, Bearsden, Bearsden Road Glasgow, Glasgow G61 1QH, UK
E-mail address: I.Ramsey@vet.gla.ac.uk

Vet Clin Small Anim 40 (2010) 269–283
doi:10.1016/j.cvsm.2009.10.008
0195-5616/10/$ – see front matter © 2010 Elsevier Inc. All rights reserved.

vetsmall.theclinics.com

17-hydroxyprogesterone, and androstenedione) (**Fig. 1**). Trilostane does not appear to have any direct hormonal activity of its own and does not interact with the main sex hormone receptors.[11]

Most studies on the mode of action of trilostane have been performed in vitro, in laboratory rats, or in humans. There is little information on the effect of trilostane in healthy dogs. In dogs with HAC, it has been shown that trilostane causes a significant increase in 17-hydroxypregnenolone and DHEA concentrations.[12] These results confirmed an inhibitory effect of trilostane on the 3β-HSD system. However, the investigators also noted that 17-hydroxyprogesterone concentrations did not change in dogs treated with trilostane despite a marked decrease in cortisol concentrations. They postulated that, in addition to its inhibitory effect on the 3β-HSD system, trilostane has an influence on 11β-hydroxylase, which would result in a reduction in the conversion of 17-hydroxyprogesterone to cortisol, and possibly on the interconversion of cortisol, and cortisone by 11β-hydroxysteroid dehydrogenase (11β-HSD).[12] However, further studies by the same group demonstrated that cortisone concentrations in normal dogs are increased by ACTH.[13] This does not consistently happen in human beings, which suggests that the 11β-HSD enzyme in dogs is subtly different from the human equivalent. In addition, cortisone concentrations in dogs with pituitary-dependent HAC (PDH) are consistently increased; again, this is in contrast to the situation in human beings.[13] Trilostane treatment reduces the concentration of cortisone (both basal and following stimulation with ACTH) in dogs with PDH, but to a lesser extent than it reduces cortisol concentrations.[13] Therefore, although trilostane may have an effect on 11β-HSD, until more is known about the canine version of this

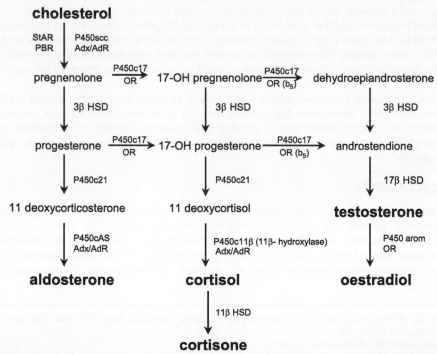

Fig. 1. Biosynthetic pathways in steroidogenesis. Different tissues of the adrenal gland express different enzymes, so not all processes occur in all cells. The principal target for the competitive inhibitor trilostane is 3β-hydroxysteroid dehydrogenase.

enzyme it is not possible to say this with any certainty. The effects of trilostane on dogs may be different to the effects on humans because steroid synthesis is subtly different between the species.

PHARMACOLOGY

Few pharmacokinetic studies have been performed on trilostane. In the rat and monkey, trilostane is rapidly absorbed after oral dosing, with peak blood concentrations occurring between 0.5 and 1 hour (rat) and between 2 and 4 hours (monkey).[14] In human volunteers, the peak concentrations were between 2 and 4 hours.[15] In dogs, peak trilostane concentrations are seen within 1.5 hours and decrease to baseline values in about 18 hours (Dechra Veterinary Products Limited, UK, unpublished data). The variability exhibited in systemic levels of trilostane after oral administration is possibly due in part to suboptimal absorption owing to its low water solubility. It has been shown that feeding immediately after the administration of trilostane increases its absorption.[16] Trilostane is cleared from the blood after 7 hours in the rat, 6 to 8 hours in the human, and 48 hours in the monkey. After the administration of trilostane to rats, the metabolite ketotrilostane is formed within a few minutes.[17] Ketotrilostane has about 1.7 times the activity of trilostane in steroid inhibition.[15] Conversely, when ketotrilostane is given to rats, trilostane is rapidly formed, suggesting that these compounds exist in equilibrium in vivo. Trilostane and ketotrilostane are metabolized into any 1 of 4 further metabolites. Excretion in rats is mainly via feces, whereas in monkeys urinary excretion is more important.[14]

USE IN CANINE PDH

The clinical use of trilostane in canine HAC, and in particular PDH, has now been evaluated in several published clinical studies from centers across the world.[18–23] In addition, unpublished studies have been conducted for regulatory purposes (Dechra Veterinary Products, unpublished data). Many other studies of the specific endocrine effects of trilostane have also been published, but insufficient clinical data are presented to assess this aspect. Direct metanalysis of the combined data from these studies is not useful because the study populations (referral or first opinion; PDH only or all HAC), diagnostic evaluations, starting doses, monitoring methods, dose adjustment protocols, and end points vary among the studies. However, comparison of these published studies is worthwhile and is summarized in **Table 1**. It should be noted that some of these studies were funded, at least in part, by commercial sources.

Starting Dose and Frequency

The starting dose of the 6 studies listed in **Table 1** ranged from 0.5 mg/kg twice daily to 20 mg/kg once daily. To some extent, the available formulations determined this choice. The finishing dose range in each study was even more variable; however, the mean/median dose was in the range 2.8 to 7.3 mg/kg in 5 of the studies (although in 2 of these studies, the dose was split twice daily). It therefore seems logical to recommend a starting dose in the range 2 to 5 mg/kg/d.

There are no studies that directly compare different frequencies of trilostane administration. Four of the studies in **Table 1** used once-daily dosing as the starting point.[18–20,23] However, it has been demonstrated that the effect of trilostane on basal and ACTH-stimulated cortisol is considerably less than 24 hours in most cases.[24] In the same study, the investigators also documented 6 dogs with HAC whose clinical signs were poorly controlled and whose post-ACTH concentrations observed 4 and 24 hours after the administration of trilostane were always higher than the equivalent

Table 1
Summary of 6 clinical studies on the use of trilostane in canine HAC

References	18	19	20	21	22	23
Country	Switzerland	United Kingdom	Australia	Spain	United States	Netherlands
Study design						
PDH dogs	11	78	30	44	18	63
ADH dogs	0	0	0	0	4	0
Starting dose	Median, 6.3 mg/kg q 24 h Range, 3.9-9.2	Mean, 5.9 mg/kg q 24 h Range, 1.8-20	Median, NS Range, 3-12	Mean, 3.1 mg/kg q 12 h (SD = 1.3)	Median, 1.4 mg/kg q 12 h Range, 0.5-2.5	Median, NS Range, 2-4 mg/kg q 24 h
Monitoring	1, 3-4, 6-7, 12-16, 24-28 wk	10 d, 4, 12, 24 wk, then every 12-24 wk	10, 30, 90, 180 d	7 d, 1, 3, 6 mo, then every 6 mo	1-2, 4-8, 8-16 wk	3 wk, then every 3 wk until stable
Target cortisol range	27-69 nmol/L	20-250 nmol/L	25-125 nmol/L	27-135 nmol/L	<150 nmol/L	30-190 nmol/L
Time of sampling	2-6 h	Most within a few hours	No particular time	4-6 h, at 7 d, then 8-12 h	3-4 h	2-4 h
Tablets given with food	Unknown	Unknown	Unknown	NS	Yes	NS
Length of follow-up	7 dogs for 1 y, 3 dogs for 2 y	Up to 4 y, 30 dogs for more than 24 wk	Mean, 384 d; range, 170-600 d	Up to 3.5 y	16 wk	Up to 12 wk
Study results						
Dose changes	4 increased and 3 decreased during study	23 increased and 9 decreased during study	NS	10 increased and 2 decreased at 1 mo	10 increased 4-8 wk 5 increased 8-16 wk	22 increased and 4 decreased during study

Withdrawals	None	None	None	None	6 dogs (4 had surgery for ADH)	None
Final dose	Median, 6.1 mg/kg q 24 h Range, 4.1–15.6 mg/kg	Mean, 7.3 mg/kg q 24 h Range, 1.6–27.2 mg/kg[a]	Median, 16.7 mg/kg q 24 h Range, 5–50 mg/kg	Mean, 3.2 mg/kg q 12 h	Mean, 1.7 mg/kg q 12 h Range, 1.1–2.8 mg/kg	Mean, 2.8 mg/kg q 24 h Range, 0.8–5.8 mg/kg
Clinical efficacy	9 (82%) improved after 6 mo of treatment	60 (77%) improved by 4 wk. 24/39 dogs with alopecia improved	30 (100%) improved at 90 d	20 stable and improved of 30 (67%) at 6 mo	15 improved at 4–8 wk, 16/18 (89%) at 8–16 wk	60 (95%) improved
Dogs in target cortisol range	Median above target range at 4 reevaluations	59 (76%) at some time during study	17 (57%) at 90 d, 23 of 29 (79%) at 180 d	26 of 36 (72%) at 3 mo	14 of 16 (87%) at 8–16 wk	100% (definition of inclusion)
Adverse effects	2 minor adverse events	2 dogs died early on hypoAC in 2 dogs (1 died). 13 other minor adverse events	1 died (unrelated cause). No others in first 6 mo, later 4 cases of hypoAC	hypoAC in 11 (25%)	hypoAC in 2 dogs	hypoAC in 5 dogs, 3 during the study and 2 after study completed
Other comments			5 dogs had failed other treatments before start of study	Mean survival time 31 mo (95% CI, 26–36)	3 dogs treated q 8 h	

Abbreviations: ADH, adrenal-dependent HAC; CI, confidence interval; NS, not stated in paper; SD, standard deviation.

[a] Figures not in article but provided by authors from original data.

cortisol concentrations in 4 dogs whose clinical signs were controlled. When 4 of the dogs with poorly controlled clinical signs were switched to twice-daily dosing, the clinical condition of 3 of them improved and their cortisol responsiveness to ACTH stimulation was reduced both after 4 and 24 hours. Following the publication of these results, 2 studies opted to start dogs on a twice-daily regimen.[21,22] However, the overall results obtained in these 2 studies were not superior to those obtained in earlier studies.[18–20] It is likely that at least a few dogs require twice-daily dosing with trilostane to achieve control; however, it is probably not necessary to divide the starting dose for all dogs. In 1 study in which trilostane was used twice daily in all dogs, there was a higher rate of adverse incidents than in any of the other 5 studies in **Table 1**.[21]

Monitoring

In the 6 studies listed in **Table 1**, the frequency of monitoring is one of the most consistent features. However, the basis for this frequency is not clear. The caution of the early studies may not be appropriate now that more is known about the response to trilostane. In particular, the clinical signs and cortisol concentrations continue to improve in most dogs in the first month.[19,20] Performing an ACTH stimulation test 10 to 14 days after starting therapy may not be so useful because changing the dose at this stage would risk increasing the dose of trilostane too early. Very few cases develop trilostane overdose in the first 2 weeks of therapy. A review consultation could be adequate, and an ACTH stimulation test only performed if adverse effects have been noted. Monthly monitoring for the first 3 months, followed by monitoring every 3 months for the first year and every 4 to 6 months thereafter may well be adequate.

Most clinical studies to date have used the clinical signs and the ACTH stimulation test as the primary methods of assessing control.[18–23] In these studies, trilostane caused significant reductions in both the mean basal and post-ACTH stimulation cortisol concentrations in dogs with HAC in the first month of treatment. Furthermore these improvements were also maintained in the study populations for the duration of the trial. However, despite its widespread use, the ACTH stimulation test has never been validated for trilostane therapy.

The ACTH stimulation test does provide a valuable assessment of the immediate capacity of the adrenal glands to secrete cortisol. For drugs (such as mitotane) and diseases (such as immune-mediated hypoadrenocorticism) that cause permanent effects on the adrenal gland, the ACTH stimulation test provides an effective method of assessing the adrenal gland. However, because of the relatively short-lasting effects of trilostane, the ACTH stimulation test varies considerably with the time of testing relative to dosing.[24] Because of the lack of this knowledge, early studies of trilostane showed clinical effects that were sometimes discordant with the ACTH stimulation test results. The short duration of action of trilostane may have a protective effect against the development of hypoadrenocorticism, as many dogs with no serum cortisol response to ACTH stimulation 2 to 3 hours post trilostane dosing do not develop signs of hypoadrenocorticism.[18] However many dogs that have a target level serum cortisol post ACTH stimulation test will exhibit signs of HAC.[20,24] Various timings and cortisol target levels have been used for the ACTH stimulation test when the test was used to monitor trilostane therapy.[18–23] The lower the target range the greater the chance of hypoadrenocorticism. However, in the earlier studies, many dogs did not have their cortisol levels reduced to the investigators' stated target range.[18–21] Later studies, which tended to be more precise on the timing of the ACTH stimulation test, achieved a higher rate of success in this respect.[22,23]

Based on the data in **Table 1**, the author's currently recommended target range for the post-ACTH cortisol concentration is 40 to 120 nmol/L (1.4–4.3 µg/dL) for ACTH stimulation tests started 2 to 4 hours after dosing; however, if dogs have a post-ACTH cortisol concentration of 120 to 200 nmol/L (4.3–7.2 μg/dL) and are responding well to treatment, then an increase in monitoring rather than dose may be more acceptable to the owners. Other methods of monitoring trilostane are under active investigation and are considered later in the article.

Dose Changes

Most of the published studies on trilostane treatment record details of the number of dose changes. To some extent, this has to be interpreted in the light of the starting dose and the target range for post-ACTH cortisol concentrations in an individual study. However, in all studies, a sizeable proportion of dogs required a dose increase and a small minority required a dose decrease. These results emphasize the importance of regular monitoring when treating a case of canine HAC. Even once-stable dogs may become unstable at subsequent monitoring visits.

Efficacy and Survival

In the studies in **Table 1**, trilostane was found to be between 67% and 100% effective in resolving the various signs of HAC over 3 to 6 months.[18–23] In contrast, mitotane is effective in about 80% of cases of PDH.[25] It is reasonable to conclude that trilostane is at least as effective as mitotane in controlling the clinical signs of most cases of canine HAC.

There have been 2 studies that have compared the survival times of dogs treated with trilostane with those treated with mitotane.[26,27] In the first study, the survival times of 148 dogs treated for PDH were studied using clinical records from 3 UK veterinary centers.[26] Of these animals, 123 (83.1%) were treated with trilostane and 25 (16.9%) were treated with mitotane. The median survival time for animals treated with trilostane was 662 days (range, 8–1971), and for mitotane it was 708 days (range, 33–1339). There was no significant difference between the survival times for animals treated with trilostane and those treated with mitotane (**Fig. 2**).

In the second study, the median survival time of 40 dogs treated with trilostane twice a day (900 days) was significantly longer ($P = .05$) than the median survival time (720 days) of 46 dogs treated with mitotane using a nonselective adrenocorticolytic protocol.[27] Both protocols had similar levels of long-term efficacy (75%), although short-term efficacy with mitotane was higher. They also had a similar prevalence of side effects (25%), although 2 of the mitotane-treated dogs died. This prevalence of side effects with trilostane has not been recorded by others.[18–23] In those countries that do not currently regard either routine twice-daily dosing with trilostane or nonselective adrenocorticolysis with mitotane as first-choice protocols, this study has more relevance to animals that have failed a conventional first-choice protocol.

Safety (to Humans)

Trilostane does not require any special safety precautions in its handling. It is formulated in capsules that are now available in a range of sizes (therefore splitting or reformulating capsules should not be necessary). If a capsule is accidentally damaged, the drug does not cross the skin barrier. Ingestion or inhalation of small quantities of trilostane would be expected to have no effect on a human being. If taken in large doses (which would have to be a deliberate action), trilostane can act as an abortifacient and could potentially induce hypocortisolism. Doses of 60 mg or more, given 4 times daily over 4 weeks, were used in 10 healthy men, with minimal effects on their adrenal function.[28] In contrast, the risks of handling mitotane are well documented.[29] Trilostane is safer than mitotane for humans to handle.

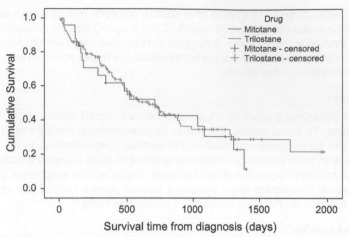

Fig. 2. Kaplan-Meier Survival Curve for mitotane- and trilostane-treated animals. Dogs alive at the completion of the study and those lost to follow-up were censored (indicated by a vertical line). (*From* Barker EN, Campbell S, Tebb AJ, et al. A comparison of the survival times of dogs treated with mitotane or trilostane for pituitary-dependent hyperadrenocorticism. J Vet Intern Med 2005;19(6):812; with permission.)

Safety and Adverse Effects in Dogs

One common feature of the studies in **Table 1** is that trilostane seems to be well tolerated by almost all dogs. If the numbers of dogs from these 6 clinical trials are combined, then only 39 of 244 dogs (16%) treated with trilostane developed adverse effects that may have been attributable to trilostane.[18–23] This prevalence of side effects compares favorably with to those reported with mitotane (25%–42%).[25,30,31]

If failure to respond is regarded as an adverse effect, then it is probably the most common adverse effect of trilostane administration. In these cases, an increase in the dose (and/or frequency) or a change to an alternative medication (such as mitotane) is indicated. More serious side effects include (in order of severity) adrenal necrosis, hypoadrenocorticism, and hyperkalemia. These side effects are described in the following sections.

Adrenal Necrosis and HAC

The most serious side effect of trilostane that has been identified to date is acute adrenal necrosis. This has been documented in 2 case reports, 1 fatal and the other requiring permanent glucocorticoid therapy.[32,33] Acute adrenal necrosis may also have been the cause of sudden death and sudden decreases in trilostane requirement in a few other cases.[16] Necrosis of the adrenal cortex cannot be directly explained by the competitive inhibition of steroidogenesis. However, adrenal necrosis also cannot be dismissed as isolated idiosyncratic reactions. Varying degrees of adrenal necrosis and associated inflammation have been described in 5 of 7 non-randomly selected postmortems of dogs that had been treated with trilostane.[34] All 7 dogs also showed some degree of adrenal hyperplasia. In 2 dogs the lesions were severe enough to have been associated with hypoadrenocorticism, however both cases had also received mitotane. In both cases and in 4 of the other dogs other causes of death were also definitively established. The severity of the lesions may have been related to the doses of trilostane used and the duration of treatment.[34] The inference from this study is that adrenal hyperplasia is common in trilostane-treated dogs, but it may also be associated with a low-grade adrenal necrosis.

The development of adrenal necrosis could be because of the hypersecretion of ACTH.[34] It has been demonstrated that trilostane causes an increase in ACTH concentrations.[35] This leads to the increase in the size of the adrenal glands that is observed in many dogs that are treated with trilostane.[36] Moreover, it has been shown that even short periods of administration of ACTH can also, paradoxically, result in degeneration, focal necrosis, and hemorrhage of human adrenal glands.[37]

Adrenal necrosis does not explain most of the cases of hypoadrenocorticism seen in trilostane-treated dogs. Most cases of hypoadrenocorticism associated with trilostane recover rapidly after temporary cessation of the drug but continue to require the drug to control the clinical signs. This suggests that these cases have suffered from overdosage rather than adrenal necrosis.[18–23] Most affected cases have electrolyte changes (hyponatremia, hyperkalemia) typical of hypoadrenocorticism. However, 1 case that developed isolated hypocortisolism has been described.[33]

There is also a theoretical risk that trilostane-induced adrenal hyperplasia could develop into adrenal tumors.[34] However, no evidence for this has been published.

ACTH concentrations also increase in normal dogs that are treated with trilostane.[38] This is associated with an increase in pituitary size (as assessed by magnetic resonance imaging) and histologic evidence of pituitary corticotroph hyperplasia and bilateral adrenal hyperplasia. It seems reasonable to assume that trilostane could result in an increase in the size of pituitary tumors, but again, no evidence for this has been published.

Hyperkalemia

Two of the 6 clinical studies in **Table 1** recorded a mild increase in median serum potassium concentrations.[18,21] Dogs that develop hyperkalemia do not appear to have a low aldosterone concentration (Ramsey and Neiger, unpublished observations, 2005). The mechanism of action of this hyperkalemia has not been identified. Any trilostane-treated dog with a mild increase in potassium should be checked with an ACTH stimulation test, rather than empirically reducing the dose. Trilostane can then be safely withheld while waiting for the results of the test.

Other Side Effects

Trilostane is associated with vomiting and diarrhea in some dogs, independently of any effects on cortisol levels. Successful treatment with trilostane might also lead to the development of previously suppressed immune-mediated, inflammatory or neoplastic diseases; however, so far, there have been no reports of these side effects. All of these effects are well described in relation to the use of mitotane, and readers are referred to standard texts for descriptions of these side effects.[25]

Use in Dogs with PDH and Concurrent Conditions

Manufacturers recommend that trilostane should not be used in animals suffering from primary hepatic disease and/or renal insufficiency. However, the basis for this recommendation is unclear in the published literature. Information is not available on what dosage adjustment should be made in dogs with primary hepatic disease and/or renal insufficiency. Similarly, there are no studies looking at trilostane use in dogs with concurrent diabetes mellitus and HAC. Currently the author does not reduce the dose of trilostane when treating a dog with diabetes and HAC. It seems logical to give trilostane and insulin at the same frequency (ie, either both once a day or both twice a day).

USE IN CANINE ADRENAL-DEPENDENT HAC

There have been no large-scale studies of the treatment of adrenal-dependent HAC (ADH) in dogs. However, trilostane does appear to work in ADH. Evidence of efficacy is provided by 1 small series and a couple of case reports.[39–41] It is not known if the dose, frequency, or monitoring of trilostane treatment in ADH cases should be the same as in PDH cases or not. Until more data are available, it would be prudent to exercise caution when using trilostane in such cases.

EFFECTS ON OTHER ENDOCRINE PARAMETERS
Effect on Aldosterone

Aldosterone secretion in dogs with untreated HAC is generally considered to be decreased.[42,43] The effect of trilostane on aldosterone secretion in dogs with HAC has been reported in 3 studies. One study of 15 dogs suggested an increase in basal plasma aldosterone concentrations (PAC) with trilostane treatment.[12] In 2 other studies (of 17 and 63 dogs), trilostane did not appear to have a significant effect on basal PAC.[23,44] Trilostane does appear to reduce ACTH-stimulated aldosterone concentrations in dogs with HAC.[12,44] A reduction in both basal and ACTH-stimulated aldosterone concentrations is also seen in mitotane-treated dogs.[42,43] In all the 3 studies, the observed effects on aldosterone concentrations were less pronounced than the effects on cortisol concentrations.

In humans, and it is suggested in dogs, plasma rennin activity (PRA) (and specifically the PRA:PAC ratio) is a better indicator of mineralocorticoid deficiency than PAC alone.[23] It has been shown in a series of 63 dogs that PRA is increased and the PRA:PAC ratio is reduced by trilostane therapy.[23]

Effect on Urinary Corticoid to Creatinine Ratio

If the ACTH stimulation test only provides a measure of the short-term effects of trilostane then there is a need to identify a test that measures the long-term control of HAC. Initially it would appear that the urinary corticoid to creatinine ratio (UCCR) makes a logical choice. However, an early study reported that it was not useful, although few details were given.[18] Another early study demonstrated that the mean UCCR did not decrease significantly with trilostane treatment.[20] The investigators of this study did, however, note that the UCCR was lower when the urine was collected shortly after dosing and higher when collected later. These investigators felt that UCCR was useful to assess the duration of effect of trilostane when collected 24 hours after dosing, when it had the least effect. However, overall correlation with ACTH stimulation test results and clinical improvement was low in this study.[20] In a recent prospective study of 18 dogs that had been successfully treated with once-daily trilostane, UCCRs were monitored every 2 weeks for at least 8 weeks.[45] Although UCCRs did decrease compared with pretreatment values, they did not fall to below the upper limit of the reference range in most dogs. Moreover, the UCCRs of 11 dogs that initially had insufficient doses of trilostane did not differ significantly from when the dosage was optimal. Post-ACTH cortisol concentrations did not correlate significantly with UCCRs at rechecks during trilostane treatment. However, UCCR could be used with greater success to identify dogs that were being overtreated with trilostane. These results are similar to those achieved with mitotane.[46–48]

However, another recent study using twice-daily trilostane suggested that measuring UCCR in a urine sample collected at home the same morning as a postdosing ACTH stimulation test was performed provided useful data with regard to the duration of effect of the trilostane.[22] In many cases, this replaces a second (predosing)

ACTH stimulation test being performed in dogs that had failed to respond to once-daily dosing as described by others.[24] Further research is needed to confirm these findings.

Effect on Haptoglobin and Other Acute Phase Proteins

Glucocorticoids have been demonstrated to cause a significant increase in hapto-globin concentrations, and haptoglobin has been assessed as a marker for good control of HAC with trilostane.[49] Although serum haptoglobin concentrations decreased with trilostane therapy, the concentrations did not closely relate to the degree of control of HAC as assessed by an ACTH stimulation test. A further study demonstrated that haptoglobin measurements, even when combined with other parameters such as cholesterol and/or alkaline phosphatase, were only moderately informative of disease control. The study also demonstrated that serum amyloid A decreased with trilostane therapy, but not C-reactive protein.[50]

Effect on Thyroid and Parathyroid Hormones

HAC is associated with a reduction in thyroxine.[51] Fourteen of 20 dogs demonstrated an increase in thyroxine after trilostane treatment; however, although the mean concentration increased, this increase was not found to be significant.[52] In contrast, there was a significant increase in the mean concentrations of thyroid-stimulating hormone, with 14 of the 20 dogs demonstrating an increase (of these 14 dogs, 10 also showed an increase in thyroxine concentrations). There was a significant decrease in the mean free thyroxine concentration (although most of the treated dogs had concentrations that were within the reference range).

HAC is also associated with an increase in parathyroid hormone concentrations, which can be regarded as adrenal secondary hyperparathyroidism.[53] Trilostane treatment has also been shown to cause a decrease in parathyroid hormone concentrations, although many dogs do not return to normal.[54]

OTHER USES OF TRILOSTANE IN DOGS

Trilostane has been demonstrated to be effective in the treatment of alopecia X in Pomeranians, poodles, and Alaskan malamutes, which many authorities consider to be a mild, slowly progressive form of PDH.[55,56] The doses used in these 2 studies were different (9–11 mg/kg once daily for the Pomeranians and miniature poodles, 3.0–3.6 mg/kg once daily for the Alaskan malamutes). Two of the Pomeranians did not respond to this dose but did respond when the dose was increased by doubling the frequency of administration to twice daily.[55] The efficacy of trilostane in alopecia X is in marked contrast to the inconsistent and often temporary results achieved with other therapies, such as melatonin, thyroxine, and sex hormones. As the condition does not usually progress rapidly or cause other significant effects (such as polyuria or polyphagia), the need for, and risks of, therapy should be carefully discussed with owners before starting trilostane.

In humans, trilostane has been used to treat human hyperaldosteronism.[6] Although the effects of trilostane on aldosterone are less than on cortisol, it would be possible to contemplate the use of trilostane in a case of canine or feline hyperaldosteronism (Conn syndrome), particularly when aldosterone antagonists such as spironolactone have not been effective.

TRILOSTANE IN HAC IN OTHER SPECIES

The use of trilostane has been reported in the treatment of cats, horses, and guinea pigs with HAC.[57–60] The drug seems to have similar effects to those described in dogs; however, data is limited and caution is advisable. One study of 5 cats with hyperadrenocorticism that were treated with trilostane reported that all 5 cats showed an improvement in their clinical signs and endocrine test results, however all continued to have some signs of hypercortisolism.[59] There were no reductions in the insulin requirements of the 3 cats in this study that were also diabetic. Two of the cats died or were euthanized after 16 and 140 days whereas 3 were still alive 6, 11 and 20 months after the start of trilostane therapy. There is 1 case report of the use of trilostane in a cat with bilateral adrenal enlargement and excessive sex steroid hormone production.[61]

SUMMARY AND FUTURE STUDIES

The introduction of trilostane has increased the options for the management of canine HAC in many countries. The drug is safer than mitotane for humans to handle; it is nearly as effective as mitotane and has a lower frequency of serious adverse reactions.

The optimal dosing interval has still to be formally determined. Studies that compare the success of once-daily with twice-daily administration will be important. Whatever the starting dose and frequency, trilostane therapy still requires careful monitoring. However, the ACTH stimulation test may be suboptimal as the only method used to assess the efficacy and safety of trilostane. Although to date, no better method has been identified, it is important that further studies are undertaken on the UCCR and other measurements of total daily cortisol production. The long-term frequency of such monitoring should also be properly assessed.

Trilostane does not cure HAC, and some cases are not well controlled by it. In these poorly controlled cases, other therapeutic options (specifically mitotane) are indicated. Therefore access to mitotane and the skills required to use it still need to be maintained within the veterinary profession.

REFERENCES

1. Neuman HC, Potts GO, Ryan WT, et al. Steroidal heterocycles XIII. 4alpha, 4-epoxy-5alpha-androst-2-eno(2,3-d)isoxazoles and related compounds (1970). J Med Chem 1970;13(5):948–51.
2. Potts GO, Creange JE, Hardomg HR, et al. Trilostane, an orally active inhibitor of steroid biosynthesis. Steroids 1978;32(2):257–67.
3. Komanicky P, Spark RF, Melby JC. Treatment of Cushing's syndrome with trilostane (WIN 24,540), an inhibitor of adrenal steroid biosynthesis. J Clin Endocrinol Metab 1978;47(5):1042–51.
4. Dewis P, Anderson DC, Bu'lock DE, et al. Experience with trilostane in the treatment of Cushing's syndrome. Clin Endocrinol (Oxf) 1983;18(6):533–40.
5. Semple CG, Beastall GH, Gray CE, et al. Trilostane in the management of Cushing's syndrome. Acta Endocrinol (Copenh) 1983;102(1):107–10.
6. Winterberg B, Vetter W, Groth H, et al. Primary aldosteronism: treatment with trilostane. Cardiology 1985;72(Suppl 1):117–21.
7. Williams CJ, Barley V, Blackledge G, et al. Multicenter study of trilostane: a new hormonal agent in advanced postmenopausal breast cancer. Cancer Treat Rep 1987;71(12):1197–201.

8. Biller BMK, Grossman AB, Stewart PM, et al. Treatment of adrenocorticotropin-dependent Cushing's syndrome: a consensus statement. J Clin Endocrinol Metab 2008;93(7):2454–62.

9. Puddefoot JR, Barker S, Vinson GP. Trilostane in advanced breast cancer. Expert Opin Pharmacother 2006;7(17):2413–9.

10. Hurley K, Sturgess K, Cauvin A, et al. The use of trilostane for the treatment of hyperadrenocorticism in dogs [abstract]. J Vet Intern Med 1998;12(3):210.

11. Tueni E, Devleeschouwer N, Leclercq G, et al. Endocrine effects of trilostane: in vitro and in vivo studies. Eur J Cancer Clin Oncol 1987;23(10):1461–7.

12. Sieber-Ruckstuhl NS, Boretti FS, Wenger M, et al. Cortisol, aldosterone, cortisol precursor, androgen and endogenous ACTH concentrations in dogs with pituitary-dependant hyperadrenocorticism treated with trilostane. Domest Anim Endocrinol 2006;31(1):63–75.

13. Sieber-Ruckstuhl NS, Boretti FS, Wenger M, et al. Serum concentrations of cortisol and cortisone in healthy dogs and dogs with pituitary-dependent hyperadrenocorticism treated with trilostane. Vet Rec 2008;163(16):477–81.

14. Baker JF, Benziger D, Chalecki BW, et al. Disposition of trilostane in the rat and monkey. Arch Int Pharmacodyn Ther 1980;243(1):4–16.

15. Robinson DT, Earnshaw RJ, Mitchell R, et al. The bioavailability and metabolism of trilostane in normal subjects, a comparative study using high pressure liquid chromatographic and quantitative cytochemical assays. J Steroid Biochem 1984;21(5):601–5.

16. Johnston L, Chohan A, Chapman E. Absorption of trilostane in the fasted and non-fasted healthy dog [abstract]. Proceedings of the 15th ECVIM Congress; 2005. p. 223.

17. McGee JP, Shaw PN. The pharmacokinetics of trilostane and ketotrilostane in an interconverting system in the rat. Pharm Res 1992;9(4):464–8.

18. Ruckstuhl NS, Nett CS, Reusch CE. Results of clinical examinations, laboratory tests, and ultrasonography in dogs with pituitary-dependent hyperadrenocorticism treated with trilostane. Am J Vet Res 2002;63(4):506–12.

19. Neiger R, Ramsey I, O'Connor J, et al. Trilostane treatment of 78 dogs with pituitary-dependent hyperadrenocorticism. Vet Rec 2002;150(26):799–804.

20. Braddock JA, Church DB, Robertson ID, et al. Trilostane treatment in dogs with pituitary-dependent hyperadrenocorticism. Aust Vet J 2003;81(10):600–7.

21. Alenza DP, Arenas C, Lopez ML, et al. Long-term efficacy of trilostane administered twice daily in dogs with pituitary-dependent hyperadrenocorticism. J Am Anim Hosp Assoc 2006;42(4):269–76.

22. Vaughan MA, Feldman EC, Hoar BR, et al. Evaluation of twice-daily, low-dose trilostane treatment administered orally in dogs with naturally occurring hyperadrenocorticism. J Am Vet Med Assoc 2008;232(9):1321–8.

23. Galac S, Buijtels JJ, Mol JA, et al. Effects of trilostane on the pituitary-adrenocortical and renin-aldosterone axis in dogs with pituitary-dependent hypercortisolism. Vet J 2008. [Epub ahead of print].

24. Bell R, Neiger R, McGrotty Y, et al. Study of the effects of once daily doses of trilostane on cortisol concentrations and responsiveness to adrenocorticotrophic hormone in hyperadrenocorticoid dogs. Vet Rec 2006;159(9):277–81.

25. Kintzer PP, Peterson ME. Mitotane (o, p-DDD) treatment of 200 dogs with pituitary-dependent hyperadrenocorticism. J Vet Intern Med 1991;5(3):182–90.

26. Barker EN, Campbell S, Tebb AJ, et al. A comparison of the survival times of dogs treated with mitotane or trilostane for pituitary-dependent hyperadrenocorticism. J Vet Intern Med 2005;19(6):810–5.

27. Clemente M, De Andrés PJ, Arenas C, et al. Comparison of non-selective adrenocorticolysis with mitotane or trilostane for the treatment of dogs with pituitary-dependent hyperadrenocorticism. Vet Rec 2007;161(24):805–9.

28. Semple CG, Thomson JA, Stark AN, et al. Trilostane and the normal hypothalamic-pituitary-adrenocortical axis. Clin Endocrinol (Oxf) 1982;17(6):569–75.

29. Feldman EC, Nelson RW. Canine hyperadrenocorticism (Cushing's syndrome). In: Canine and feline endocrinology and reproduction. 3rd edition. Philadelphia: Saunders; 2004. p. 252–357.

30. Lorenz MD. Diagnosis and medical management of canine Cushing's syndrome: a study of 57 consecutive cases. J Am Anim Hosp Assoc 1982;18(5):707–16.

31. Dunn KJ, Herrtage ME, Dunn JK. Use of ACTH stimulation tests to monitor the treatment of canine hyperadrenocorticism. Vet Rec 1995;137(7):161–5.

32. Chapman PS, Kelly DF, Archer J, et al. Adrenal necrosis in a dog receiving trilostane for the treatment of hyperadrenocorticism. J Small Anim Pract 2004;45(6):307–10.

33. Ramsey IK, Richardson J, Lenard Z, et al. Persistent isolated hypocortisolism following brief treatment with trilostane. Aust Vet J 2008;86(12):491–5.

34. Reusch CE, Sieber-Ruckstuhl N, Wenger M, et al. Histological evaluation of the adrenal glands of seven dogs with hyperadrenocorticism treated with trilostane. Vet Rec 2007;160(7):219–24.

35. Witt AL, Neiger R. Adrenocorticotropic hormone levels in dogs with pituitary-dependent hyperadrenocorticism following trilostane therapy. Vet Rec 2004; 154(13):399–400.

36. Mantis P, Lamb CR, Witt AL, et al. Changes in ultrasonographic appearance of adrenal glands in dogs with pituitary-dependent hyperadrenocorticism treated with trilostane. Vet Radiol Ultrasound 2003;44(6):682–5.

37. Wilbur OM Jr, Riach AR. A study of the role of adrenocorticotrophic hormone (ACTH) in the pathogenesis of tubular degeneration of the adrenals. Bull John Hopkins Hosp 1953;93(5):321–47.

38. Teshima T, Hara Y, Takekoshi S, et al. Trilostane-induced inhibition of cortisol secretion results in reduced negative feedback at the hypothalamic-pituitary axis. Domest Anim Endocrinol 2009;36(1):32–44.

39. Eastwood JM, Elwood CM, Hurley KJ. Trilostane treatment of a dog with functional adrenocortical neoplasia. J Small Anim Pract 2003;44(3):126–31.

40. Benchekroun G, de Fornel-Thibaud P, Lafarge S, et al. Trilostane therapy for hyperadrenocorticism in three dogs with adrenocortical metastasis. Vet Rec 2008; 163(6):190–2.

41. Machida T, Uchida E, Matsuda K, et al. Aldosterone-, corticosterone- and cortisol-secreting adrenocortical carcinoma in a dog: case report. J Vet Med Sci 2008;70(3):317–20.

42. Golden DL, Lothrop CD Jr. A retrospective study of aldosterone secretion in normal and adrenopathic dogs. J Vet Intern Med 1988;2(3):121–5.

43. Goy-Thollot I, Péchereau D, Kéroack S, et al. Investigation of the role of aldosterone in hypertension associated with spontaneous pituitary-dependent hyperadrenocorticism in dogs. J Small Anim Pract 2002;43(11):489–92.

44. Wenger M, Sieber-Ruckstuhl NS, Müller C, et al. Effect of trilostane on serum concentrations of aldosterone, cortisol, and potassium in dogs with pituitary-dependent hyperadrenocorticism. Am J Vet Res 2004;65(9):1245–50 [Erratum in: Am J Vet Res 2004;65(11):1562].

45. Galac S, Buijtels JJ, Kooistra HS. Urinary corticoid: creatinine ratios in dogs with pituitary-dependent hypercortisolism during trilostane treatment. J Vet Intern Med 2009. [Epub ahead of print].

46. Randolph JF, Toomey J, Center SA, et al. Use of the urine cortisol-to-creatinine ratio for monitoring dogs with pituitary-dependent hyperadrenocorticism during induction treatment with mitotane (o, p'-DDD). Am J Vet Res 1998;59(3):258–61.

47. Angles JM, Feldman EC, Nelson RW, et al. Use of urine cortisol:creatinine ratio versus adrenocorticotropic hormone stimulation testing for monitoring mitotane treatment of pituitary-dependent hyperadrenocorticism in dogs. J Am Vet Med Assoc 1997;211(8):1002–4.

48. Guptill L, Scott-Moncrieff JC, Bottoms G, et al. Use of the urine cortisol: creatinine ratio to monitor treatment response in dogs with pituitary-dependent hyperadrenocorticism. J Am Vet Med Assoc 1997;210(8):1158–61.

49. McGrotty YL, Arteaga A, Knottenbelt CM, et al. Haptoglobin concentrations in dogs undergoing trilostane treatment for hyperadrenocorticism. Vet Clin Pathol 2005;34(3):255–8.

50. Arteaga A, Dhand NK, McCann T, et al. Monitoring the response of canine hyperadrenocorticism to trilostane treatment assessing acute phase protein concentrations. J Small Anim Pract, in press.

51. Peterson ME, Ferguson DC, Kintzer PP, et al. Effects of spontaneous hyperadrenocorticism on serum thyroid hormone concentrations in the dog. Am J Vet Res 1984;45(10):2034–8.

52. Kenefick SJ, Neiger R. The effect of trilostane treatment on circulating thyroid hormone concentrations in dogs with pituitary-dependent hyperadrenocorticism. J Small Anim Pract 2008;49(3):139–43.

53. Ramsey IK, Tebb A, Harris E, et al. Hyperparathyroidism in dogs with hyperadrenocorticism. J Small Anim Pract 2005;46(11):531–6.

54. Tebb AJ, Arteaga A, Evans H, et al. Canine hyperadrenocorticism: effects of trilostane on parathyroid hormone, calcium and phosphate concentrations. J Small Anim Pract 2005;46(11):537–42.

55. Cerundolo R, Lloyd DH, Persechino A, et al. Treatment of canine Alopecia X with trilostane. Vet Dermatol 2004;15(5):285–93.

56. Leone F, Cerundolo R, Vercelli A, et al. The use of trilostane for the treatment of alopecia X in Alaskan malamutes. J Am Anim Hosp Assoc 2005;41(5):336–42.

57. McGowan CM, Neiger R. Efficacy of trilostane for the treatment of equine Cushing's syndrome. Equine Vet J 2003;35(4):414–8.

58. Skelly BJ, Petrus D, Nicholls PK. Use of trilostane for the treatment of pituitary-dependent hyperadrenocorticism in a cat. J Small Anim Pract 2003;44(6):269–72.

59. Neiger R, Witt AL, Noble A, et al. Trilostane therapy for treatment of pituitary-dependent hyperadrenocorticism in 5 cats. J Vet Intern Med 2004;18(2):160–4.

60. Zeugswetter F, Fenske M, Hassan J, et al. Cushing's syndrome in a guinea pig. Vet Rec 2007;160(25):878–80.

61. Boag AK, Neiger R, Church DB. Trilostane treatment of bilateral adrenal enlargement and excessive sex steroid hormone production in a cat. J Small Anim Pract 2004;45(5):263–6.

46. Panciera DL, Cooper SA, et al. Use of the urine cortisol-to-creatinine ratio for monitoring dogs with pituitary-dependent hyperadrenocorticism treated with trilostane. J Am Vet Med Assoc 230 (2007) 258-61.

47. Ramsey IK, Tebb A, Herrtage ME, et al. Use of low-dose intradermal ACTH stimulation testing for monitoring treatment of canine spontaneous hyperadrenocorticism in dogs. J Am Vet Med Assoc 198 (1991) 1214.

48. Galac S, Buijtels JJ, Mol JA, et al. Effect of trilostane on the pituitary-adrenocortical and renin-aldosterone axis in dogs with pituitary-dependent hyperadrenocorticism. J Am Vet Med Assoc 155-6.

49. McGrotty YL, Arteaga A, Knottenbelt CM, et al. Unpredictable cortisol slope in dogs undergoing trilostane treatment for hyperadrenocorticism. Vet Clin Pathol 39 (2010) 281.

50. Arteaga A, Dhand NK, McCann T, et al. Monitoring the response of canine hyperadrenocorticism to trilostane treatment assessed by pre-pill plasma cortisol concentrations. J Small Anim Pract (in press).

51. Peterson ME, Ferguson DC, Kintzer PP, et al. Effects of spontaneous hyperadrenocorticism on serum iodine concentration in the dog. Am J Vet Res 29 (1984) 2034-6.

52. Benitah N, Feldman EC, Kass PH, et al. The effect of trilostane treatment on thyroid hormone concentrations in dogs with pituitary-dependent hyperadrenocorticism. J Small Anim Pract 50 (2009) 138-46.

53. Ramsey IK, Tebb A, Harris E, et al. Hypoadrenocorticism in dogs with hyperadrenocorticism. J Small Anim Pract 2005; 46 (7) 531-6.

54. Tebb AJ, Arteaga A, Evans H, et al. Canine hyperadrenocorticism: effects of trilostane on parathyroid hormone, calcium and phosphate concentrations. J Small Anim Pract 2007; 48 (11) 537-42.

55. Greco DS, Harpold LM, et al. Treatment of adult-onset primary hypoadrenocorticism. Vet Clin North Am Small Anim Pract 31 (2001) 1233-41.

56. Gallelli MF, Cabrera-Blatter MF, et al. The use of trilostane for the treatment of spontaneous hyperadrenocorticism in a dog. J Am Anim Hosp Assoc 2009; 45 (2) 123-6.

57. McGowan CM, Neiger R. Efficacy of trilostane for the treatment of equine Cushing's syndrome. Equine Vet J 2003; 35 (4) 414-8.

58. Greco DS, Peterson ME. Use of trilostane for the treatment of primary hyperadrenocorticism in a cat. J Small Anim Pract 2001; 42 (9) 449-72.

59. Neiger R, Witt AL, Noble A, et al. Trilostane therapy for treatment of pituitary-dependent hyperadrenocorticism in 5 cats. J Vet Intern Med 2004; 18 (2) 160-4.

60. Zadro-Weber I, Ferebee M, Hassan TA, et al. Cushing's syndrome in feline patients. J Vet Res 2007; 160 (23) 919-90.

61. Greco AR, Neiger R, Charron DB. Trilostane treatment of mineralocorticoid replacement and excessive sex steroid hormone production in a cat. J Small Anim Pract 2003; 44 (5) 439-3.

Atypical Cushing's Syndrome in Dogs: Arguments For and Against

Ellen N. Behrend, VMD, PhD*, Robert Kennis, DVM, MS

KEYWORDS

- Hyperadrenocorticism • Sex hormones • Cushing's syndrome
- Adrenal gland • Alopecia X

Hyperadrenocorticism (HAC), also known as Cushing's syndrome, is one of the most common, if not the most common, endocrinopathies of older dogs. Due to the high incidence and relatively nonspecific clinical signs, older dogs are commonly screened for HAC. Diagnosis requires testing with the low-dose dexamethasone suppression test (LDDST) or the standard corticotropin (ACTH) stimulation test with measurement of serum cortisol pre- and post-ACTH injection.[1] Unfortunately, neither test is perfect, however.

To understand how good a test is, comprehension of the statistical terms *sensitivity* and *specificity* is helpful. Sensitivity is the percentage of individuals with the disease who are correctly identified by the test. For example, if the LDDST is 95% sensitive for diagnosing HAC, then of all dogs with the disease, 95% would have abnormal LDDST results consistent with HAC and the other 5% would not. Specificity is the percentage of individuals without the disease who have a negative result. For example, if the ACTH stimulation test has a specificity of 86% for diagnosing HAC, then, of all dogs with positive ACTH stimulation test results, 86% would have the disease and 14% would have a false-positive result.

For diagnosing HAC, the LDDST offers a sensitivity of approximately 95%, while the ACTH stimulation test offers a sensitivity of approximately 80%. For pituitary-dependent HAC (PDH) alone, the sensitivity of the ACTH stimulation test is 87%. Meanwhile, for HAC due to adrenal tumor alone, the sensitivity of the ACTH stimulation test is 61.3%.[1] The specificity of the LDDST has been estimated to be 44% to 73%[2–5]; for the ACTH stimulation test, specificity is 64% to 86% (**Table 1**).[2,6] Since HAC occurs in older dogs, patients tested for HAC often have concurrent disease. If they do not have HAC, they at least have a nonadrenal illness causing the clinical signs. In general, the more severe the nonadrenal illness present, the more likely a false-positive test result for HAC.[2]

Department of Clinical Sciences, College of Veterinary Medicine, Auburn University, Auburn, AL 36849, USA
* Corresponding author.
E-mail address: behreen@auburn.edu (E.N. Behrend).

Vet Clin Small Anim 40 (2010) 285–296
doi:10.1016/j.cvsm.2009.11.002
0195-5616/10/$ – see front matter © 2010 Elsevier Inc. All rights reserved.

Table 1 Summary of reported sensitivities and specificities of adrenocortical function tests in dogs				
	Test			
	LDDST		ACTH Stimulation	
Condition	Sensitivity	Specificity	Sensitivity	Specificity
HAC	95%[1]	44%–73%[2–5]	80%[1]	64%–86%[2,6]
PDH	Not determined	Not determined	87%[1]	Not determined
Adrenal tumor	Not determined	Not determined	61%[1]	Not determined
Occult HAC	Not applicable	Not applicable	Not determined	70%[a,7,8]

[a] Determined only for 17OHP.

Due to imprecision of the tests, HAC can be a difficult diagnosis to make at times. Clinicians are faced with the situation where their clinical impressions are that patients have HAC, but the tests performed do not confirm the diagnosis and no alternative diagnosis is identified. Recently, to explain such circumstances, much interest has focused on a syndrome termed *occult HAC*. Dogs with occult HAC allegedly have clinical signs and/or routine laboratory abnormalities consistent with classic HAC but have normal serum cortisol concentrations on LDDST and/or ACTH stimulation tests. *Alopecia X* has been used to describe dogs with occult HAC with dermatologic changes only, mainly bilaterally symmetric alopecia and hyperpigmentation with a puppy coat (**Fig. 1**). Alopecia X is commonly seen in the Nordic breeds, Pomeranians, and chow chows, which may exhibit a telogen-predominant hair cycle with seasonal shedding.[9] In theory, occult HAC is caused by diversion of the normal adrenocortical pathways for cortisol and aldosterone synthesis into overproduction of sex hormones instead (**Fig. 2**). The syndrome is diagnosed by an ACTH stimulation test with measurement of serum sex hormones (ie, androstenedione, estradiol, progesterone, and 17-hydroxy-progesterone [17OHP]) and aldosterone concentrations pre- and post-ACTH.

However, in these authors' opinion, conclusive evidence for the existence of occult HAC as a sex hormone–mediated condition is lacking. Here we evaluate the evidence both for and against. In evaluating adrenal secretion of sex hormone and cortisol precursors (eg, 11-deoxycortisol) in dogs, it must be taken into account whether basal or ACTH-stimulated concentrations were measured. For the diagnosis of standard HAC, determination of basal cortisol concentration is not reliable and never used by

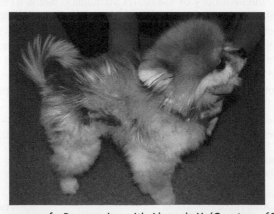

Fig. 1. Typical appearance of a Pomeranian with Alopecia X. (*Courtesy of* Dr Randy Thomas.)

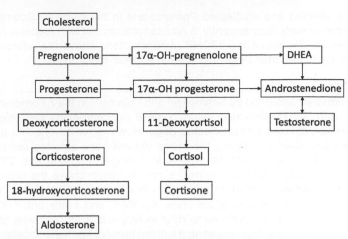

Fig. 2. The adrenocortical hormone synthesis pathway. (*Courtesy of* Dr Lauren Reid.)

itself.[1,10] No evidence has shown that measurement of basal serum sex hormone concentrations are any more reliable for diagnosis of adrenal dysfunction; thus, the following discussion will focus on ACTH-stimulated concentrations, which are a measure of adrenal reserve.

ADRENAL SEX HORMONE AND CORTISOL PRECURSOR SECRETION AS A CAUSE OF BILATERALLY SYMMETRIC ALOPECIA
Evidence in Favor

Sex hormones secreted from sources other than the adrenal glands can cause alopecia. A syndrome of castration-responsive alopecia has been recognized. Hyperestrogenism as well as hyperprogesteronism[11] associated with Sertoli cell tumors, for example, can lead to bilaterally symmetric alopecia. Administration of estrogen for treatment of urinary incontinence has led to bilaterally symmetric alopecia and histopathological changes consistent with endocrine alopecia.[12]

The first report of clinical signs thought to be due to elevations in adrenal-derived sex hormone concentrations described diffuse bilaterally symmetric alopecia and hyperpigmentation in seven Pomeranians.[13] Classic HAC was ruled out on the basis of normal ACTH stimulation test and LDDST results. Progesterone, 17OHP, 11-deoxycortisol, dehydroepiandrosterone sulfate (DHEAS), testosterone, androstenedione, and estradiol were measured pre- and post-ACTH in 7 affected Pomeranians, 12 unaffected Pomeranians, and 19 non-Pomeranian control dogs. Only ACTH-stimulated 17OHP concentrations were different between affected and unaffected Pomeranians, but ACTH-stimulated progesterone and DHEAS concentrations were significantly higher in both affected and unaffected Pomeranians as compared with the controls. Given the constellation of abnormalities in both affected and unaffected Pomeranians, Schmeitzel and Lothrop[13] hypothesized the alopecia was due to a partial deficiency of 21-hydroxylase, an enzyme needed for cortisol synthesis. In humans with 21-hydroxylase deficiency and resultant congenital adrenal hyperplasia, cortisol is not synthesized and cortisol precursors, most notably 17OHP and androgens, accumulate.[14] Because affected Pomeranians had normal serum cortisol concentrations, the enzyme deficiency was assumed to be partial.[13] Family members of people with congenital adrenal hyperplasia have sex hormone elevations to a lesser magnitude and no clinical signs, thus explaining the abnormalities in the unaffected Pomeranians (many of the affected and unaffected Pomeranians in the study by Schmeitzel and Lothrop[13] were related). Subsequently, 3 Alaskan malamutes with Alopecia X were reported to have ACTH-stimulated 17OHP concentrations above the reference range and significantly higher than those in 3 normal Alaskan malamutes.[15]

Evidence Against

Of six sex hormones assessed by Schmeitzel and Lothrop[13] in the 7 Pomeranians with Alopecia X, only ACTH-stimulated serum 17OHP concentrations were significantly different between affected and unaffected dogs. However, when affected males and females were assessed separately, the males did not have elevated serum 17OHP concentrations. In 276 dogs with Alopecia X, including 63 Pomeranians, 73% had at least one basal or post-ACTH sex hormone concentration above the normal range. Despite the preponderance of elevations in sex hormone concentrations, though, no consistent sex hormone abnormalities were identified, and Frank and colleagues[16] concluded that it is more appropriate to refer to Alopecia X as "alopecia associated with follicular arrest" rather than equating it with an adrenal hormone imbalance.

Due to the postulation by Schmeitzel and Lothrop[13] that the alopecia in Pomeranians was due to partial 21-hydroxylase deficiency, Takada and colleagues[17] cloned the canine 21-hydroxylase gene and evaluated genetic polymorphisms. No mutations affecting the primary structure of the enzyme or gene expression were identified.

Assessment

Although 21-hydroxylase abnormalities were not documented in dogs with Alopecia X,[17] another enzyme could be involved. Abnormalities of other enzymes in the cortisol synthesis pathway have been documented to cause congenital adrenal hyperplasia in people.[14] To date, however, no search for genes outside of the cortisol synthesis pathway has been successful either.[18,19] More importantly, sex hormone abnormalities appear to be easily documented in dogs with Alopecia X, but no correlation exists between elevations in any hormone and a clinical abnormality. Sex hormones are no longer believed to be related to Alopecia X.

17-HYDROXY-PROGESTERONE, OTHER SEX HORMONES, AND CORTISOL PRECURSORS AS CAUSES OF OCCULT HYPERADRENOCORTICISM
Evidence in Favor

A study of 23 dogs with clinical and routine laboratory findings suggestive of HAC was reported recently. Of the 23 dogs, 11 assigned to group 1 had typical HAC with elevated cortisol responses to ACTH. Of 10 dogs with normal ACTH response test results, 6 had positive LDDST results (group 2A), 4 had negative LDDST results (group 2B), and 3 had low plasma cortisol concentrations throughout testing (group 2C). Despite the variation in serum cortisol concentrations on the tests for standard HAC, all 23 dogs had elevated ACTH-stimulated 17OHP concentrations. Thus, Ristic and colleagues[20] concluded that ACTH-stimulated serum 17OHP concentration is elevated in dogs with classic as well as occult HAC and measurement of serum 17OHP concentrations is a marker of adrenal dysfunction.

Numerous other studies have also documented elevations in sex hormone concentrations in dogs with various forms of hypercortisolemia, either PDH or adrenal tumor. In 11 dogs with hypercortisolemia, ACTH-stimulated DHEAS was elevated in 4 of 9, androstenedione was elevated in 7 of 10, progesterone was elevated in 11 of 11, and 17OHP concentrations were elevated in 6 of 11. No dog had elevated ACTH-stimulated testosterone concentrations.[21] In 14 dogs with PDH, at least 6 and as many as 9 had elevated ACTH-stimulated 17α-hydroxypregnenolone, 17OHP,

21-deoxycortisol, or 11-deoxycortisol concentrations.[22] Of dogs with suspected HAC and elevated ACTH-stimulated serum cortisol concentrations, 71% of 59 had elevated ACTH-stimulated 17OHP and 60% of 53 had elevated corticosterone concentrations.[7] In 9 dogs with cortisol-secreting adrenal carcinoma and 10 dogs with PDH, 1 or more had elevations in serum ACTH-stimulated androstenedione, progesterone, 17OHP, testosterone, or estradiol concentrations.[23] Lastly, in 53 dogs with confirmed HAC, 69% had elevated ACTH-stimulated 17OHP concentrations. An additional 2 dogs had elevated 17OHP concentrations despite normal cortisol concentrations on both the ACTH stimulation test and LDDST. One of those 2 dogs had confirmed occult HAC based on response to mitotane. In the other, the diagnosis of occult HAC was not verified.[24]

More specifically to the point, in cases in which cortisol and sex hormones are both elevated, determining which hormones are causing clinical signs of HAC is difficult or impossible. However, sporadic reports exist of dogs with sex hormone–secreting adrenal tumors and low serum cortisol concentrations but in which clinical signs of HAC were present, ostensibly due to the sex hormones. Two dogs with adrenal tumors had clinical signs of HAC despite markedly suppressed ACTH-stimulated serum cortisol concentrations. One tumor secreted progesterone, 17OHP, testosterone, and DHEAS, while the other secreted androstenedione, estradiol, progesterone, and 17OHP.[25] In a report of eight dogs with adrenal tumor and signs of HAC, three had suppressed ACTH-stimulated serum cortisol concentrations and one had elevated 17OHP concentrations; no other sex hormones were measured in any dog nor in the other two with subnormal cortisol concentrations.[26]

Evidence Against

It is difficult to understand how sex hormones would cause clinical signs of HAC. The sex hormone most mentioned as a cause of occult HAC is progesterone. Due to progesterone's short half-life, however, little is known about the effects of elevated serum concentrations. Chronic excesses in progesterone concentration are not unique. In estrus and diestrus, serum progesterone is elevated for 60 to 90 days and often approaches or exceeds 50 to 100 times anestrus concentrations, yet no clinical signs of HAC develop.[10] In humans, clinically silent 17OHP-secreting adrenal tumors occur.[27,28] Massive elevations in serum 17OHP occur with 21-hydroxylase deficiency in people, yet clinically affected patients show signs either of aldosterone deficiency or androgen excess.[14,29] Clinical signs of HAC do not occur despite 17OHP concentrations ranging from 3000 to 40,000 ng/dL (reference range 20–600) in people.[29] Lastly, a "cryptic" syndrome of 21-hydroxylase deficiency exists in which affected people lack 21-hydroxylase and have hormonal abnormalities but no clinical signs. The factors that impose the phenotypic variability on the genotypic abnormality are unknown,[29] but abnormal sex hormone elevations by themselves are not sufficient to cause clinical disease. Similarly, in dogs with Alopecia X, serum 17OHP concentrations can be quite elevated, similar to what is seen with dogs with purported occult HAC, yet none of the classical systemic clinical signs, such as polyuria/polydipsia, polyphagia, pot belly, and panting, are reported.

Two mechanisms have been proposed for progesterone's ability to cause signs of glucocorticoid excess. Synthetic progestins, compounds with progesterone-like actions, may either bind glucocorticoid receptors[30] or may displace cortisol from its binding protein, thereby elevating serum free cortisol concentrations.[31] Indeed, progestins suppress endogenous ACTH secretion and cause adrenal atrophy, an action suggestive of glucocorticoid activity.[32–34] Accordingly, progesterone may do the same. Examination of Pomeranians with Alopecia X, however, refutes the likelihood of either mechanism occurring. If elevated serum 17OHP concentration, as seen in those dogs, is sufficient to cause clinical disease due to glucocorticoid actions of 17OHP, endogenous ACTH concentration should be suppressed because of negative feedback effects of glucocorticoids on the pituitary. Indeed, for dogs with proven sex hormone–secreting tumors and signs of HAC despite hypocortisolemia, measured endogenous ACTH concentrations were low.[25] However, not all dogs with clinical signs supposedly due to sex hormones have suppression of ACTH secretion.[13] To the contrary, Pomeranians with elevated serum 17OHP concentrations had higher plasma ACTH concentrations than did healthy dogs.[13] Similarly, during diestrus, when serum progesterone concentrations are highest, adrenal secretion of cortisol in response to ACTH is greatest.[35] Lastly, in the report of eight dogs with adrenal tumor, another dog had elevated ACTH-stimulated 17OHP concentrations, but cortisol secretion was not suppressed.

How adrenal tumor could have a shift in hormone synthesis activity can be understood easily. Tumor cells are not normal and can undergo loss of differentiation, losing the ability to synthesize enzymes in the hormone synthesis pathways. In cases of pituitary-dependent occult HAC, how or why normal adrenocortical tissue should alter steroid synthesis is unexplained.

The number of published cases of dogs with purported true occult HAC (ie, presence of consistent clinical signs, ACTH stimulation test and LDDST both normal, and response to appropriate therapy) is actually quite small. Problems exist with the initial study that attributed occult HAC to elevated 17OHP concentration.[20] Classifying all 23 dogs as having occult HAC was inappropriate because 17 had standard ACTH stimulation test or LDDST results consistent with HAC and were not occult. Three dogs had normal ACTH stimulation test results and low plasma cortisol concentrations throughout the LDDST. These results are not unusual in dogs with an adrenal tumor. Only 3 dogs were diagnosed with PDH despite having both normal ACTH stimulation test and LDDST results.[20] In 64 dogs documented to have HAC, no dog was negative on both the ACTH stimulation test and LDDST.[36] Out of 57 dogs evaluated recently for HAC with cortisol measurements on a ACTH stimulation test and LDDST, 40 were diagnosed as having PDH, 12 as having adrenal tumor, and 5 as possibly having occult HAC. The diagnosis of occult HAC was bolstered by a positive response to therapy in only 1 dog in the latter group, suggesting that only 1 of 57 dogs may have had occult HAC.[24]

Assessment

Sex hormone concentrations have been reportedly elevated in dogs with either PDH or adrenal tumors. In most cases, it is impossible to tell whether excess cortisol or sex hormones are causing the clinical signs. Sex hormone elevations, however, have been documented to cause clinical signs of HAC even in cases in which cortisol concentrations are suppressed. On the other hand, in humans, sex hormone elevations either cause no clinical signs or signs associated with the reproductive function of the hormones, but never signs of occult HAC. A mechanism by which sex hormones could cause the signs of occult HAC, or by which adrenal glands could shift their hormone production in PDH, is lacking. Occult HAC, if it does exist, has been possibly documented in only a handful of cases.

SEX HORMONE PANEL TESTING
Evidence in Favor

Measurement of serum sex hormone concentrations has been advocated as a means of diagnosing occult HAC. Use of a panel of hormones has been stated to increase sensitivity and specificity of the test over measurement of a single hormone alone.[37] Elevations in concentrations of any hormone can be common, with estradiol elevations noted in approximately 40% of panels submitted to one reference laboratory.[37]

Evidence Against

Unfortunately, sensitivity and specificity of adrenal sex hormone panel testing have not been published in a peer-reviewed journal. Neither have elevations in sex hormone concentrations been evaluated in the context of occult HAC, as was done for Alopecia X; although sex hormones previously were believed to cause Alopecia X, retrospective analysis of sex hormone panel results identified the abnormalities as coincidental and not causative.[16]

The specificity of sex hormone panel testing must be considered. It is reasonable to assume that dogs with nonadrenal illness (eg, a dog with diabetes mellitus) might not have the same ACTH response as healthy dogs because of adaptation of adrenocortical function to the stresses of chronic illness.[6] Indeed, two landmark studies assessed the response to ACTH in dogs not suspected to have HAC but that did have nonadrenal illness,[2,6] and their results revolutionized how ACTH stimulation test results are evaluated. Many stressed and sick dogs have increased cortisol concentrations and an exaggerated ACTH response, but do not have HAC. Dogs with chronic nonadrenal illness had a 14%[2] or 36%[6] chance of having ACTH stimulation test results consistent with HAC. In other words, if testing a dog with nonadrenal illness to see if it also has HAC, a dog with an ACTH stimulation test result consistent with HAC still has up to a 36% chance of not having HAC! Similarly, if chronic nonadrenal illness is present and causing clinical signs similar to those of HAC even though HAC is not present, a positive ACTH stimulation test may yield a false diagnosis of HAC in up to one-third of patients and the real disease may be missed.

As such, the likelihood that activation of the pituitary-adrenal axis in nonadrenal illness would also cause a shift toward synthesis and secretion of sex hormones is unknown. In one study, post-ACTH serum cortisol, 17OHP, and corticosterone concentrations were significantly correlated both in dogs with neoplasia and those suspected of having HAC, suggesting that as adrenal function is increased either by adrenal disease or nonspecifically by nonadrenal illness, production of all hormones increases proportionately.[7]

With regard to 17OHP, the specificity of the test may be as low as 70% (ie, the chance of a false-positive result is 30%) (see Table 1).[7,8] In one study of 35 dogs with neoplasia but without adrenal disease, 30% had elevated serum 17OHP concentrations post-ACTH stimulation.[7] When dogs suspected to have HAC but proven not to were compared with those that did have HAC, cortisol distinguished the two groups more clearly than did either 17α-hydroxypregnenolone[22] or 17OHP.[8,22] In 30% of dogs suspected to have HAC but for which alternate diagnoses were found, serum ACTH-stimulated 17OHP concentrations were elevated.[8] Thus, if 17OHP were measured to make the diagnosis in a similar population of dogs, 30% would be mistakenly misdiagnosed as having HAC. In 6 dogs with either pheochromocytoma or a nonfunctional adrenal tumor, concentrations of androstenedione, progesterone, 17OHP, testosterone, or estradiol were elevated in all.[23] Therefore, dogs without adrenal disease clearly can have elevated sex hormone concentrations as they do cortisol concentrations, and sex hormones may be more likely to be falsely elevated by nonadrenal illness as compared with cortisol.

Unfortunately, the ability of chronic nonadrenal illness to affect sex hormone testing has not received critical appraisal as has the ability of chronic nonadrenal illness to affect the standard ACTH stimulation test. Besides 17OHP, other sex hormones measured to diagnose occult HAC include basal and ACTH-stimulated estradiol, progesterone, testosterone, and androstenedione. However, the accuracy of this test remains to be determined.

Assessment

Numerous dogs have been documented to have elevated sex hormone concentrations with signs of occult HAC, but the association between hormone abnormalities and the clinical signs has not undergone rigorous assessment. Similarly, the specificity of adrenal sex hormone panel testing has not been evaluated. Elevations at least in serum ACTH-stimulated 17OHP concentrations apparently are more often due to nonadrenal illness than to cortisol.

RESPONSE TO TREATMENT
Evidence in Favor

In dogs with either Alopecia X or purported occult HAC, treatment with agents that affect pituitary or adrenal function has resulted in resolution of clinical signs. Melatonin is a neurohormone produced by the pineal gland, which controls seasonal reproductive and hair growth cycles and alters sex hormone concentrations in intact dogs.[38] In 29 dogs with Alopecia X, melatonin was administered initially at 3 mg/kg every 12 hours to dogs weighing 15 kg or less, and 6 mg/kg every 12 hours to dogs weighing more than 15 kg.[39] Dogs were reevaluated approximately every 4 months and, based on clinical response, melatonin therapy was continued at the same or at an increased dose (if ≤15 kg, 4.5 mg every 12 hours; if >15 kg, 9–12 mg every 12 hours), or therapy was switched to mitotane, an adrenocorticolytic agent with preference for the adrenal zonae reticulata and fasicularis, the zones that secrete cortisol and sex hormones (25 mg/kg orally daily or divided twice daily for 5–7 days followed by 25 mg/kg orally divided twice weekly). Of the 29 dogs, 15 had partial hair regrowth at first reevaluation.[39] In 3 Alaskan malamutes with Alopecia X, treatment with trilostane (3.0–3.6 mg/kg daily by mouth), a drug that inhibits the adrenal enzyme 3β-hydroxysteroid dehydrogenase and inhibits adrenal hormone synthesis,[40] resulted in complete hair regrowth within 6 months.[15] Of 16 Pomeranians and 8 miniature poodles with Alopecia X, 14 Pomeranians and all poodles had hair regrowth in response to trilostane; the mean dose that caused hair regrowth was 11.8 mg/kg (range 5–23.5) in Pomeranians and 9 mg/kg (range 6.1–15.0) per day in the poodles.[41] In the study on occult HAC by Ristic and colleagues,[20] 9 dogs in groups 2A, B, or C (ie, were diagnosed with HAC but had normal ACTH-stimulated cortisol concentrations) were treated with trilostane or mitotane, and all had clinical improvement. Decreased ACTH-stimulated cortisol or 17OHP concentrations were documented in 4 of the 9. Lastly, in 1 dog with clinical signs of HAC and normal post–ACTH-stimulated cortisol and LDDST results but an elevated ACTH-stimulated 17OHP concentration, clinical signs resolved with mitotane therapy.[24]

Evidence Against

The response to mitotane, melatonin, or trilostane has not been uniform or predictable. In 15 Pomeranians with Alopecia X, melatonin (mean 1.3 mg/kg by mouth twice a day; range 1.0–1.7) for 3 months, only 6 (40%) had mild to moderate hair regrowth.[42] In the study evaluating 29 dogs that were diagnosed with Alopecia X and treated with melatonin or mitotane, partial or complete hair regrowth was seen in only 62% overall. After the first recheck, melatonin dosage was increased in 8 dogs, but only 1 had improved hair growth. On mitotane, 4 of 6 dogs had partial to complete hair regrowth and 2 had none.[39] More importantly, serum sex hormone concentrations did not change significantly in response to treatment nor correlate with whether response was seen. Of the dogs with partial or complete hair regrowth, androstenedione was still elevated in 21%, progesterone was still elevated in 64%, and 17OHP was still elevated in 36%.[39] In 16 Pomeranians and 8 miniature poodles with Alopecia X that responded to trilostane therapy, 17OHP concentrations were significantly elevated by therapy.[41] Similarly, 2 dogs with occult HAC treated with trilostane had clinical signs resolve despite 17OHP concentrations being higher with therapy.[20] Thus, hair coat and other clinical signs improve despite further increases in concentrations of the sex hormones purportedly underlying the clinical signs.

Assessment

Although successful therapy has been reported, three main problems exist. First, not all dogs respond to melatonin, mitotane, or trilostane. Second, response does not correlate with sex hormone concentrations. Hair regrowth can occur even in dogs in which serum sex hormone concentrations do not improve. Third, serum sex hormone concentrations can even increase while the clinical signs resolve. If the sex hormones are causing the clinical signs, it is hard to explain how lack of change or even further elevations in sex hormones can be associated with remission if the sex hormones are causing the clinical signs.

SUMMARY

Occult HAC due to adrenal secretion of sex hormones has never been proven. In the literature, both human and veterinary, evidence exists both in favor and against the theory. Using the research into Alopecia X as an analogy for occult HAC, although occult HAC was originally thought to be due to sex hormone abnormalities, and although elevations in sex hormone concentrations were widely documented in dogs with Alopecia X, later research was unable to correlate elevations in any hormone with a clinical abnormality. The specificity of adrenal sex hormone panel testing needs to be carefully evaluated because evidence suggests that nonadrenal illness may commonly and nonspecifically increase sex hormone concentrations. Furthermore, not all dogs diagnosed with occult HAC respond to therapy directed at minimizing adrenal hormone secretion. Sex hormones may be elevated even further by therapy, yet dogs may improve clinically.

The possibility remains that "occult HAC" may exist as a syndrome, but one that is not caused by sex hormone secretion. Given the response of some cases of Alopecia X to therapy directed at hormone secretion, it is possible that local factors, such as enzymes, growth factors, or hormone receptors, may contribute to the hair cycle abnormalities and be acted upon by substances secreted by the adrenal glands to manifest the clinical signs. The same could be true of occult HAC. For example, abnormal local tissue response to cortisol could cause the syndrome. Alternatively, occult HAC may represent the canine form of metabolic syndrome as seen in people and horses. Much work remains to be done to understand both the adrenal and local tissue contribution to the syndrome of occult HAC.

REFERENCES

1. Behrend EN, Kemppainen RJ. Diagnosis of canine hyperadrenocorticism. Vet Clin North Am Small Anim Pract 2001;31:985–1003.

2. Kaplan AJ, Peterson ME, Kemppainen RJ. Effects of disease on the results of diagnostic tests for use in detecting hyperadrenocorticism in dogs. J Am Vet Med Assoc 1995;207:445–51.

3. van Liew CH, Greco DS, Salman MD. Comparison of results of adrenocorticotropic hormone stimulation and low-dose dexamethasone suppression test with necropsy findings in dogs: 81 cases (1985–1995). J Am Vet Med Assoc 1997; 211:322–5.

4. Zerbe CA. Screening tests to diagnose hyperadrenocorticism in cats and dogs. Compend Contin Educ Vet 2000;22:17–31.

5. Rijnberk A, van Wees A, Mol JA. Assessment of two tests for the diagnosis of canine hyperadrenocorticism. Vet Rec 1988;122:178–80.

6. Chastain CB, Franklin RT, Ganjam VK, et al. Evaluation of the hypothalamic pituitary-adrenal axis in clinically stressed dogs. J Am Anim Hosp Assoc 1986;22: 435–42.

7. Behrend EN, Kemppainen RJ, Boozer AL, et al. Serum 17-α-hydroxyprogesterone and corticosterone concentrations in dogs with non-adrenal neoplasia and dogs with suspected hyperadrenocorticism. J Am Vet Med Assoc 2005;227: 1762–7.

8. Chapman PS, Mooney CT, Ede J, et al. Evaluation of the basal and post-adrenocorticotrophic hormone serum concentrations of 17-hydroxyprogesterone for the diagnosis of hyperadrenocorticism in dogs. Vet Rec 2003;153:771–5.

9. Dunstan RW. A common sense approach to the morphology of the hair follicle— readdressing points of follicular confusion. 24th Proceedings of the North American Veterinary Dermatology Forum. 2009. p. 3–25.

10. Feldman EC, Nelson RW. Canine hyperadrenocorticism (Cushing's syndrome). In: Feldman EC, Nelson RW, editors. Canine and feline endocrinology and reproduction. 3rd edition. St. Louis (MO): Saunders; 2004. p. 252–357.

11. Fadok VA, Lothrop CD, Coulson P. Hyperprogestronemia associated with sertoli cell tumor and alopecia in a dog. J Am Vet Med Assoc 1986;188:1058–9.

12. Watson ADJ. Oestrogen-induced alopecia in a bitch. J Small Anim Pract 1985;26: 17–21.

13. Schmeitzel LP, Lothrop CD. Hormonal abnormalities in Pomeranians with normal coat and in Pomeranians with growth hormone–responsive dermatosis. J Am Vet Med Assoc 1990;197:1333–41.

14. Stewart PM. The adrenal cortex. In: Kronenberg HM, Melmed S, Polonsky KS, et al, editors. William's textbook of endocrinology. 11th edition. Philadelphia: Saunders Elsevier; 2008. p. 445–537.

15. Leone F, Cerundolo R, Vercelli A, et al. The use of trilostane for the treatment of alopecia X in Alaskan malamutes. J Am Anim Hosp Assoc 2005;41:336–42.

16. Frank LA, Hnilica KA, Rohrbach BW, et al. Retrospective evaluation of sex hormones and steroid hormone intermediates in dogs with alopecia. Vet Dermatol 2003;14:91–7.

17. Takada K, Kitamura H, Takiguchi M, et al. Cloning of canine 21-hydroxylase gene and its polymorphic analysis as a candidate gene for congenital adrenal hyperplasia-like syndrome in Pomeranians. Res Vet Sci 2002;73:159–63.

18. Mausberg E-M, Drogemuller C, Leeb T. Evaluation of the CTSL2 gene as a candidate gene for alopecia X in Pomeranians and Keeshonden. Anim Biotechnol 2007;18:291–6.

19. Mausberg E-M, Drogemuller C, Dolf G, et al. Exclusion of patched homolog 2 (PTCH2) as a candidate gene for alopecia X in Pomeranians and keeshonden. Vet Rec 2008;163:121–3.

20. Ristic JME, Ramsey IK, Heath FM, et al. The use of 17-hydroxyprogesterone in the diagnosis of canine hyperadrenocorticism. J Vet Intern Med 2002;16:433–9.
21. Frank LA, Schmeitzel LP, Oliver J. Steroidogenic response of adrenal tissues after administration of ACTH to dogs with hypercortisolemia. J Am Vet Med Assoc 2001;218:214–6.
22. Sieber-Ruckstuhl N, Boretti FS, Wenger M, et al. Evaluation of cortisol precursors for the diagnosis of pituitary-dependent hypercortisolism in dogs. Vet Rec 2008; 162:673–8.
23. Hill KE, Scott-Moncrieff JCR, Koshko M, et al. Secretion of sex hormones in dogs with adrenal dysfunction. J Am Vet Med Assoc 2005;226:556–61.
24. Benitah N, Feldman EC, Kass PH, et al. Evaluation of serum 17-hydroxyproges-terone concentration after administration of ACTH in dogs with hyperadrenocor-ticism. J Am Vet Med Assoc 2005;227:1095–101.
25. Syme HM, Scott-Moncrieff JCR, Treadwell NG, et al. Hyperadrenocorticism asso-ciated with excessive sex hormone production by an adrenocortical tumor in two dogs. J Am Vet Med Assoc 2001;219:1725–8.
26. Norman EJ, Thompson H, Mooney CT. Dynamic adrenal function testing in eight dogs with hyperadrenocorticism associated with adrenocortical neoplasia. Vet Rec 1999;144:551–4.
27. Turton DB, O'Brian JT, Shakir KMM. Incidental adrenal nodules: association with exaggerated 17-hydroxyprogesterone response to adrenocorticotropic hormone. J Endocrinol Invest 1992;15:789–96.
28. Bondanelli M, Campo M, Trasforini G, et al. Evaluation of hormonal function in a series of incidentally discovered adrenal masses. Metabolism 1997;46: 107–13.
29. Grumbach MM, Conte FA. Disorders of sex differentiation. In: Wilson JD, Foster DW, Kronenberg HM, et al, editors. Williams textbook of endocrinology. 9th edition. Philadelphia: W.B. Saunders Company; 1998. p. 1303–425.
30. Selman PJ, Mol JA, Rutteman GR, et al. Effects of progestin administration on the hypothalamic-pituitary-adrenal axis and glucose homeostasis in dogs. J Reprod Fertil Suppl 1997;51:345–54.
31. Juchem M, Pollow K. Binding oral contraceptive progestogens to serum proteins and cytoplasmic receptor. Am J Obstet Gynecol 1990;163:2171–83.
32. Selman PJ, Mol JA, Rutteman GR, et al. Progestin treatment in the dog II. Effects on the hypothalamic-pituitary-adrenocortical axis. Eur J Endocrinol 1994;131: 422–30.
33. Court EA, Watson ADJ, Church DB, et al. Effects of delmadinone acetate on pituitary-adrenal function, glucose tolerance and growth hormone in male dogs. Aust Vet J 1998;76:555–60.
34. van den Broek AHM, O'Farrell V. Suppression of adrenocortical function in dogs receiving therapeutic doses of megestrol acetate. J Small Anim Pract 1994;35: 285–8.
35. Reimers TJ, Mummery LK, Mc Cann JP, et al. Effects of reproductive state on concentrations of thyroxine, 3,5,3′-triiodothyronine and cortisol in serum of dogs. Biol Reprod 1984;31:148–54.
36. Feldman EC. Comparison of ACTH response and dexamethasone suppression as screening tests in canine hyperadrenocorticism. J Am Vet Med Assoc 1983; 182:506–10.
37. Oliver J. Steroid profiles in the diagnosis of canine adrenal disorders. In: Annual conference proceedings of 25th American College of Veterinary Internal Medi-cine Forum. Seattle, WA; 2007. p. 471–3.

38. Ashley PF, Frank LA, Schmeitzel LP, et al. Effect of oral melatonin administration on sex hormone, prolactin and thyroid hormone concentrations in normal dogs. J Am Vet Med Assoc 1999;215:1111–5.

39. Frank LA, Hnilica KA, Oliver JW. Adrenal steroid hormone concentrations in dogs with hair cycle arrest (alopecia X) before and during treatment with melatonin and mitotane. Vet Dermatol 2004;15:278–84.

40. Sieber-Ruckstuhl NS, Boretti FS, Wenger M, et al. Cortisol, aldosterone, cortisol precursor, androgen and endogenous ACTH concentrations in dogs with pituitary-dependent hyperadrenocorticism treated with trilostane. Domest Anim Endocrinol 2006;31:63–75.

41. Cerundolo R, Lloyd DH, Persechino A, et al. Treatment of canine alopecia X with trilostane. Vet Dermatol 2004;15:285–93.

42. Frank LA, Donnell RL, Kania SA. Oestrogen receptor evaluation in Pomeranian dogs with hair cycle arrest (alopecia X) on melatonin supplementation. Vet Dermatol 2006;17:252–8.

Synthetic Insulin Analogs and Their Use in Dogs and Cats

Chen Gilor, DVM, Thomas K. Graves, DVM, PhD*

KEYWORDS

• Diabetes • Insulin analogs • Cats • Dogs

Insulin analogs are artificially altered forms of insulin that differ from native insulin but retain its physiologic effects. Recombinant insulin analogs have revolutionized insulin therapy in human diabetes mellitus, and are having an impact on diabetes treatment in veterinary patients also. Understanding the basics of insulin pharmacology and physiology, briefly reviewed here, is key to understanding the properties of synthetic insulin analogs and the rationale for their use. This article also provides an introduction to insulin analogs used in the treatment of human diabetes mellitus, and presents current knowledge on the use of insulin analogs in dogs and cats.

INSULIN PHYSIOLOGY

Insulin is secreted by the beta cells of the islets of Langerhans in the pancreas. It reaches the liver through the portal circulation and then spreads to the rest of the body and reaches its other target organs, mainly skeletal muscle and adipose tissue. Insulin synthesis and secretion are stimulated predominantly by increases in blood glucose concentrations, but the degree to which beta cells respond to glucose is modified by a multitude of other factors including nutrients, hormones, and neural input.[1]

Endogenous insulin secretion can be divided into two phases: the basal phase, in which insulin is secreted continuously at a relatively constant rate, and the bolus phase, in which insulin is secreted in response to nutrients.[2] The primary role of basal insulin secretion is to limit lipolysis and hepatic glucose production in the fasting state. Postprandial insulin primarily suppresses hepatic glucose output and stimulates glucose use by muscle, thus preventing hyperglycemia after meals.[2] Postprandial blood glucose concentration is also largely determined by other factors such as the carbohydrate, fat, and protein content of the meal, gastrointestinal transit time, and the effects of glucagon.[2] In health, insulin secretion is adjusted constantly to work in concert with these other factors to maintain euglycemia. In the war against diabetes,

Department of Veterinary Clinical Medicine, College of Veterinary Medicine, University of Illinois at Urbana-Champaign, Urbana, IL 61802, USA
* Corresponding author.
E-mail address: tgraves@illinois.edu (T.K. Graves).

Vet Clin Small Anim 40 (2010) 297–307
doi:10.1016/j.cvsm.2009.11.001
0195-5616/10/$ – see front matter © 2010 Elsevier Inc. All rights reserved.

mimicking this highly dynamic process with subcutaneous injections of insulin is a battle best fought with advanced weapons.

PHARMACOLOGY OF INSULIN ANALOGS

There is a large body of evidence indicating that tight glycemic control is essential to prevent long-term complications of human diabetes.[3–5] Intensive treatment protocols to achieve that goal often are associated with adverse effects such as hypoglycemia and undesired weight gain. The ideal insulin therapy should mimic the physiology of insulin secretion as closely as possible. In veterinary medicine, there is no clearly established benefit of tight control of blood glucose in the normal range, and the standard of care is alleviation of clinical signs while minimizing adverse effects, rather than achieving sustained euglycemia.

Insulin has a natural tendency to crystallize and precipitate, especially in the presence of zinc. In the pancreatic beta cells, insulin is stored as hexamers surrounding molecules of zinc. Insulin hexamers are slow to penetrate capillaries, but when released from the beta cells, the zinc is diluted, and hexamers are broken down to dimers and monomers that are absorbed into the blood stream.[6] In older insulin formulations, the tendency of insulin to crystallize is enhanced by modifying the solution (eg, adding zinc or protamine), thus causing precipitation in the vial and at the site of injection.[6,7] Once injected subcutaneously, the zinc is slowly diluted (and protamine slowly degraded), thus releasing insulin into the blood. This strategy has an obvious disadvantage in that insulin has to be resuspended evenly before being drawn into a syringe, which can lead to inaccuracy in dosing.[8] A second disadvantage is that the de-precipitation in the injection site is highly variable and unpredictable, and that can lead to considerable variation in insulin absorption.[2,6] Third, the older insulin formulations such as lente and neutral protamine Hagedorn (NPH) have action profiles that are inadequate when trying to mimic normal insulin secretion physiology in people with diabetes. The onsets of action are too slow, and durations of action are too long to mimic the bolus phase; at the same time, insulin action profiles are often too peaked, and durations are usually not long enough to mimic basal secretion.[2,6,9] A similar problem exists in diabetic dogs and cats. For the typical diabetic pet, twice-daily injections of insulin at mealtime are the standard of care. Using intermediate-acting insulin formulations, this protocol usually is geared toward alleviating clinical signs of diabetes. Achieving tight glycemic control is difficult and increases the risk of hypoglycemia.

Another disadvantage of treatment with traditional insulin formulations is loss of normal liver:periphery insulin concentration gradients.[10,11] Inhibition of hepatic glucose output, a major factor in maintaining euglycemia, requires high insulin concentrations in the blood, while inhibition of lipolysis requires much lower concentrations. More than half of the insulin secreted by the pancreas is removed from the bloodstream by the liver before the remainder is circulated to other target organs. When insulin is injected subcutaneously, equal concentrations are delivered to the liver, muscles, and adipose tissue. This accomplishes either appropriate control of hepatic glucose output with inappropriately high concentrations of insulin in adipose tissue (promoting weight gain), or insufficient control of hepatic glucose output leading to poor glycemic control. A synthetic insulin analog that is preferentially targeted to the liver likely would decrease the magnitude of this problem.

Synthetic insulin analogs were designed to mimic physiologic insulin secretion as closely as possible. Intensive insulin therapy protocols in people typically consist of a bolus insulin with rapid absorption and ultrashort action given at meal time, and a basal insulin given once daily.[9] These insulin analogs were designed to have more predictable action profiles than older insulin formulations, an important feature in prevention of hypoglycemic events. The synthetic insulin analogs are based on human-recombinant insulin, and are altered biochemically to change their pharmacologic properties. Amino acid substitutions in the B26–B30 region alter the tendency of insulin to crystallize while retaining the ability to activate insulin receptors.[7] All available insulin analogs are supplied as clear solutions and do not need to be resuspended before use. This reduces inaccuracy in dosing, but insulin analogs still can form hexamers at the site of injection, resulting in some degree of variability in absorption.

Insulin has a mitogenic effect in the body. This effect is mediated by the insulin receptor and the IGF-1 receptor.[12] The mitogenic effect of synthetic insulin analogs has been investigated because the modifications to their sequence change their affinity for receptors. Changes in the absolute affinity, as well as the relative affinity to the insulin receptor compared with the insulin-like growth factor (IGF)-1 receptor, might increase the mitogenicity of a synthetic analog. Few and inconsistent data exist showing increased risk of developing cancer in people treated with insulin glargine.[13,14] Contradictory evidence, however, together with obvious benefits of using insulin glargine, have led to the present consensus to support the use of insulin glargine in people with diabetes.[12,15–17] No clinical data exist regarding the mitogenicity of insulin detemir, but one experimental study suggests that it is no more mitogenic than human insulin.[18] The affinity of insulin for insulin receptors has been reported in cats and in dogs.[19–21] IGF-1 receptor affinity has been reported in dogs, but not to the authors' knowledge in cats.[22] The authors are aware of one report of affinity of an experimental synthetic insulin analog for the insulin receptor in dogs, but they know of no such reports in cats, nor have they seen reports of receptor binding studies using commercially available insulin analogs in dogs or cats.[8] As such, there is no evidence to support a claim that any insulin product (natural or synthetic) is safer than another from a mitogenesis standpoint in cats and dogs.

RAPID-ACTING INSULIN ANALOGS: LISPRO, ASPART, AND GLULISINE

Historically, a combination of regular insulin and an intermediate-acting insulin was used to replace postprandial insulin in people with diabetes. The action profile of regular insulin after subcutaneous injection, however, may be inadequate for the treatment of diabetes, because its absorption is relatively slow. Additionally, the duration of action is too long (about 5 to 8 hours in people, about 5 hours in cats and dogs).[23–25] Insulin lispro (**Fig. 1**) was the first rapid-acting analog to be approved for use in people.[7] The amino acid sequence of insulin lispro consists of a reversal of proline at the B28 position and lysine at the B29 position. This small change greatly decreases the tendency for association and enhances the rate of absorption. In people, this results in an early onset of action (30 minutes to 1 hour), a relatively high peak in activity, and a short duration of action (2 to 3 hours). Thus, subcutaneous insulin lispro is more suited to mimic postprandial insulin secretion than subcutaneous regular insulin.[7]

In insulin aspart, the praline residue at B28 is replaced with an aspartic acid residue. In insulin glulisine, lysine at B29 is replaced by glutamic acid, and on position B3, asparagine is replaced by lysine. Insulin aspart and insulin glulisine have pharmacokinetic and pharmacodynamic profiles similar to insulin lispro.[7] All three are used in people with type 1 and type 2 diabetes. In type 1 diabetics, these insulin analogs have a clear advantage over regular insulin in reducing the risk of hypoglycemic

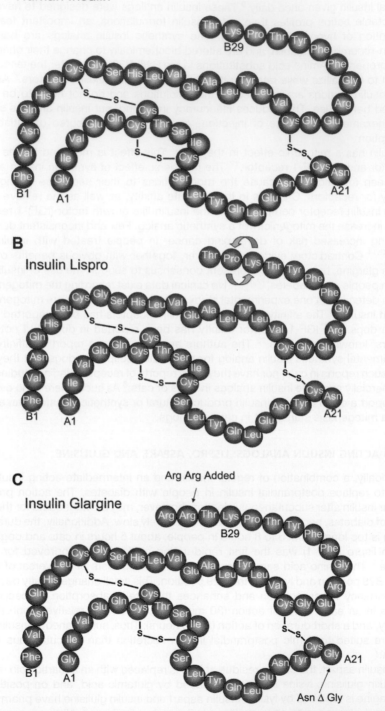

Fig. 1. Illustration of the amino acid sequences of human insulin (*A*) and three insulin analogs. In insulin lispro (*B*), the positions of proline and lysine at B28 and B29 are reversed. Insulin glargine (*C*) has glycine substituted for asparagine at A21, and two arginine residues are added to the end of the B chain. In insulin detemir (*D*), threonine at B30 is replaced with a myristic acid residue.

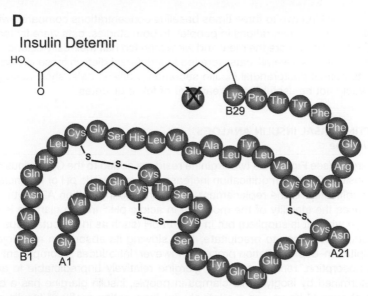

D

Insulin Detemir

Fig. 1. (*continued*)

events.[26] In type 2 diabetics, when combined with basal insulin, these analogs provide better glycemic control than regular insulin without increasing hypoglycemic episodes.[27] In one study of people with diabetes, similar glycemic control was achieved whether insulin aspart was injected 15 minutes before or 15 minutes after initiation of a meal.[28]

There are currently no reports on the use of rapid-acting analogs in the chronic treatment of diabetes in cats and dogs. Insulin lispro has been used successfully in dogs to treat diabetic ketoacidosis.[29] In that study, insulin lispro was administered intravenously and had similar efficacy as the traditionally used regular insulin. No adverse reactions were seen. There is no clear rationale for preferring insulin lispro over regular insulin for use in constant-rate intravenous insulin infusions. The biochemical alteration in insulin lispro confers greater dissociation and faster absorption of insulin injected subcutaneously, but both insulin lispro and regular insulin should dissociate immediately when delivered intravenously. This has been observed experimentally in people but not to the authors' knowledge in veterinary patients.[30] Insulin lispro also has been used experimentally in dogs in one study. It was injected once subcutaneously at a dose of 0.2 U/kg. Its plasma concentration peaked at 45 minutes and was still high at 3 hours (no further measurements were done). Insulin lispro caused a nadir in blood glucose 2 hours after injection, and the duration of action was over 3 hours.[31] Insulin aspart pharmacology also has been studied in dogs, and it was reported to have more rapid absorption following subcutaneous injection than regular insulin. The pharmacokinetics and pharmacodynamics, however, were largely similar to regular insulin.[24] The authors are aware of no reports on insulin glulisine in cats or dogs.

Rapid-acting insulin analogs were designed to replace normal bolus phase insulin secretion in people and have a duration of action of 3 hours or less. But what is the normal postprandial insulin secretion profile in dogs and cats? In two studies in non-diabetic cats, bolus phase insulin secretion had a longer duration (over 6 hours in one study and over 12 in the other) than the bolus phase in people.[32,33] The peak insulin concentration occurred later and was of lesser magnitude (occurring at 2 to

6 hours and reaching two to three times baseline concentrations compared with over five times baseline concentrations in people). In both studies, cats were fasted (overnight or for 36 hours) before the meal and were then fed half their daily caloric average over 15 to 30 minutes. Overall, cats were fed four different diets in those two studies. If this reflects normal postprandial insulin secretion profile in cats, short-acting insulin analogs would not be useful in the treatment of feline diabetes.

LONG-ACTING BASAL INSULIN ANALOGS
Insulin Glargine

Insulin glargine (see **Fig. 1**) has two arginine residues added to the C-terminus of the B chain at position 30. This modification increases the isoelectric pH of the molecule. A second modification is the replacement of asparagine in position A21 with glycine. This increases the stability of the molecule in acidic pH.[2] Insulin glargine is soluble at pH 4.0 (in which it is supplied) but in neutral pH (such as in subcutaneous tissue), it has a strong tendency to precipitate, thus slowing its absorption after injection.[8] The precipitation–deprecipitation process, however, introduces a component of variability in absorption, rendering insulin glargine relatively unpredictable in action.[34] When determined by isoglycemic clamps in people, insulin glargine has a duration of action of over 24 hours and a relatively flat time–action profile.[34] Insulin glargine is commonly used in people as once-daily basal insulin therapy, often supplemented with ultrashort-acting insulin analogs given at meal time. Compared with the traditional intermediate-acting formulations, insulin glargine offers similar reductions in glycosylated hemoglobin concentration but with decreased risk of hypoglycemia and greater convenience.[35–37]

In a small experimental study, the pharmacodynamics of insulin glargine have been studied in dogs and compared with NPH.[38] Using the isoglycemic clamp technique and with a dose of 0.5 U/kg, insulin glargine had a duration of action of about 18 to 24 hours with a pronounced peak at 7 hours. NPH had a shorter duration of action (about 12 hours) and peaked at 5 hours. Unexpectedly, insulin glargine had greater intersubject variability compared with NPH.

In one study of newly diagnosed diabetic cats, eight of eight cats became insulin-independent when treated with twice-a-day insulin glargine and an ultralow carbohydrate diet.[39] This remission rate was higher than the remission rate for cats treated with protamine zinc and iletin (PZI) (three of eight) and lente (two of eight) in the same study. The duration of illness before inclusion in the study was not mentioned, and the allocation into treatment groups was not random. Also, treatment protocols were not identical between groups. Lower remission rates were reported in another study, in which the goal of treatment was achieving euglycemia.[40] In this study, 84% of cats that were started on a treatment protocol (insulin glargine and intensive home monitoring of blood glucose) within 6 months of diagnosis achieved remission, while only 35% of cats that were started on the protocol after more than 6 months from diagnosis achieved remission. All cats in this study were fed an ultralow carbohydrate diet. These remission rates are similar to the results of another study in which cats treated with various insulin formulations other than insulin glargine (mostly PZI) had 68% remission rate when fed a low-carbohydrate diet.[41] Diabetes had been diagnosed recently (within 45 days) in only 11 of 31 cats in this study, but there were no differences in remission rates between those cats and others that had been diabetic for more than 45 days.

In a small clinical study in cats, once-a-day insulin glargine was compared with twice-a-day lente in cats fed an ultralow carbohydrate diet.[42] In that study, both treatment groups experienced improvement in serum fructosamine concentrations, and 16-hour blood glucose curves were improved. Four of the 13 cats of this study experienced remission of diabetes, but only one of these was in the insulin glargine-treated group. Disease duration was not presented clearly in this study. The same group of investigators reported another study in which cats with diabetes were treated with insulin glargine and fed a high-protein/low-carbohydrate diet or a control diet.[43] Both groups had improved glycemic control, but only 2 of 12 cats, 1 in each group, achieved remission. Taken together, these studies suggest that a low-carbohydrate diet in combination with glargine or any other insulin formulation is clinically useful in treating diabetes in cats. In newly diagnosed diabetic cats, treatment with glargine might be more likely to achieve remission.

INSULIN DETEMIR

In contrast to insulin glargine, pharmacodynamics of insulin detemir (see **Fig. 1**) are considered highly predictable in people, with minimal inter- and intrasubject variability.[34,44] Insulin detemir has a myristic acid residue (14-carbon fatty acid) replacing threonine at position B30. Instead of the natural, weaker, ionic interactions between insulin molecules, insulin detemir molecules associate through strong hydrophobic interactions between the fatty acids. These fatty acids also bind reversibly to albumin, which buffers the concentration of insulin detemir in the blood and tissues, adding to its protracted and more predictable effect.[6] Predictable pharmacodynamics, demonstrated with insulin detemir in human clinical trials, are key to minimizing hypoglycemic events.[34-37] The interaction of insulin detemir with albumin also increases the availability of insulin detemir to organs with fenestrated capillaries such as the liver. Relatively high concentrations of insulin detemir are achieved in the liver compared with other target tissues. Thus insulin detemir inhibits hepatic glucose output more effectively; lipogenesis in adipose tissue is decreased, and weight gain is minimized.[11,35-37,45] Other acylated long-acting insulin analogs have been described but are not in clinical use. Two of these—NN344 and O346—have been studied in dogs. O346 bound so avidly to albumin that its duration of action was approximately 2 days in dogs.[46,47] A thyroxyl–insulin analog that binds to thyroid hormone-binding proteins also has been described.[48,49] This insulin analog was hepato-selective in people and in dogs, but its duration of action in people was slightly shorter than the duration of action of NPH.

When determined by isoglycemic clamps in people, insulin detemir has a duration of action of approximately 20 hours, and it is used commonly as a once-daily basal insulin in people with diabetes.[34] Although seldom compared side by side, the clinical outcomes of treatment with insulin detemir or insulin glargine are similar. Use of these analogs is associated with similar reductions in glycosylated hemoglobin, with decreased numbers of hypoglycemic events. Insulin glargine may be slightly more effective in reducing glycosylated hemoglobin, and hypoglycemic events may be less common with the use of insulin detemir. Insulin detemir, however, consistently is associated with less undesired weight gain in people.[35-37]

INSULIN DETEMIR VERSUS INSULIN GLARGINE IN CATS

In a study in healthy cats, the duration of action of insulin glargine after a single subcutaneous injection at a dose of 0.5 U/kg was found to be 22 plus or minus 1.8 hours.[50] This was based, however, on the return of blood glucose to baseline concentrations during prolonged fasting. Although this method of studying insulin pharmacokinetics and pharmacodynamics is common in veterinary research, results of such studies may not be completely relevant, because they do not take into account endogenous insulin and normal physiologic responses to changes in blood glucose. For these reasons, studies of insulin pharmacology are better done by clamping blood glucose concentrations to euglycemia and measuring other indicators of insulin activity. The effects of prolonged fasting also were not taken into account in that study, and it is possible that the duration of action of insulin glargine was overestimated. Interestingly, in the same study, serum insulin concentrations returned to baseline within 6.7 plus or minus 1.3 hours (range 0.6 to 13 hours). The authors have compared the pharmacodynamics of single 0.5 U/kg injections of insulin detemir and insulin glargine in cats using the isoglycemic clamp method.[51] The onset of action of insulin detemir was 1.8 plus or minus 0.8 hours; the end-of action was reached at 13.5 plus or minus 3.5 hours, and there was a significant variation in the time–action profile between cats. Surprisingly, the duration of action of insulin glargine was much shorter than previously reported (11.3 plus or minus 4.5 hours), and like insulin detemir, there was a significant variation in the time–action profile between cats, ranging from curves that where essentially flat to others that had pronounced peaks.

Insulin detemir has been compared with insulin glargine in one clinical study in which the goal of treatment was tight glycemic control (maintaining euglycemia with blood glucose concentrations ranging between 50 and 100 mg/dL).[52] Blood glucose concentrations were monitored by owners at home, and the doses of insulin were changed by the owners. All cats in this study were fed high-protein/low-carbohydrate canned diets. Overall remission rates in this study were 67% for insulin detemir and 64% for insulin glargine. Hypoglycemia was common, but clinical signs rarely were noticed. Also rare was the occurrence of Somogyi effect. The median maximum insulin glargine dose was 2.5 IU (range 1.0 to 9.0 IU) compared with a median insulin detemir dose of 1.75 IU (range 0.5 to 4.0 IU). In this study, a twice-daily regimen of insulin administration was used for both analogs.

REFERENCES

1. Ahren B, Taborsky GJ. Beta-cell function and insulin secretion. In: Porte DJ, Sherwin RS, Baron A, editors. Ellenberg & Rifkin's diabetis mellitus. 6th edition. New York: McGraw-Hill Companies Inc; 2003. p. 43–65.
2. Owens DR, Bolli GB. Beyond the era of NPH insulin–long-acting insulin analogs: chemistry, comparative pharmacology, and clinical application. Diabetes Technol Ther 2008;10:333–49.
3. Nathan DM, Cleary PA, Backlund JY, et al. Intensive diabetes treatment and cardiovascular disease in patients with type 1 diabetes. N Engl J Med 2005; 353:2643–53.
4. Genuth S. Insights from the diabetes control and complications trial/epidemiology of diabetes interventions and complications study on the use of intensive glycemic treatment to reduce the risk of complications of type 1 diabetes. Endocr Pract 2006;12(Suppl 1):34–41.
5. Akalin S, Berntorp K, Ceriello A, et al. Intensive glucose therapy and clinical implications of recent data: a consensus statement from the Global Task Force on Glycaemic Control. Int J Clin Pract 2009;63:1421–5.
6. Havelund S, Plum A, Ribel U, et al. The mechanism of protraction of insulin detemir, a long-acting, acylated analog of human insulin. Pharm Res 2004;21:1498–504.
7. Sheldon B, Russell-Jones D, Wright J. Insulin analogues: an example of applied medical science. Diabetes Obes Metab 2009;11:5–19.

8. Kohn WD, Micanovic R, Myers SL, et al. pI-shifted insulin analogs with extended in vivo time action and favorable receptor selectivity. Peptides 2007;28:935–48.
9. Choe C, Edelman S. New therapeutic options for treating type-2 diabetes: a review of insulin analogs and premixed insulin analogs. J Natl Med Assoc 2007;99:357–60, 363–7.
10. Hordern SV, Wright JE, Umpleby AM, et al. Comparison of the effects on glucose and lipid metabolism of equipotent doses of insulin detemir and NPH insulin with a 16-h euglycaemic clamp. Diabetologia 2005;48:420–6.
11. Hermansen K, Davies M. Does insulin detemir have a role in reducing risk of insulin-associated weight gain? Diabetes Obes Metab 2007;9:209–17.
12. Smith U, Gale EA. Does diabetes therapy influence the risk of cancer? Diabetologia 2009;52:1699–708.
13. Weinstein D, Simon M, Yehezkel E, et al. Insulin analogues display IGF-I-like mitogenic and anti-apoptotic activities in cultured cancer cells. Diabetes Metab Res Rev 2009;25:41–9.
14. Hemkens LG, Grouven U, Bender R, et al. Risk of malignancies in patients with diabetes treated with human insulin or insulin analogues: a cohort study. Diabetologia 2009;52:1732–44.
15. Rosenstock J, Fonseca V, McGill JB, et al. Similar risk of malignancy with insulin glargine and neutral protamine Hagedorn (NPH) insulin in patients with type 2 diabetes: findings from a 5-year randomised, open-label study. Diabetologia 2009;52:1971–3.
16. Home PD, Lagarenne P. Combined randomised controlled trial experience of malignancies in studies using insulin glargine. Diabetologia 2009;52:2499–506.
17. Colhoun HM. Use of insulin glargine and cancer incidence in Scotland: a study from the Scottish Diabetes Research Network Epidemiology Group. Diabetologia 2009;52:1755–65.
18. Kurtzhals P, Schaffer L, Sorensen A, et al. Correlations of receptor binding and metabolic and mitogenic potencies of insulin analogs designed for clinical use. Diabetes 2000;49:999–1005.
19. Paxton R, Ye LX. Purification and characterization of a feline hepatic insulin receptor. Am J Vet Res 2000;61:1625–32.
20. Tolan I, Ragoobirsingh D, Morrison EY. The effect of capsaicin on blood glucose, plasma insulin levels, and insulin binding in dog models. Phytother Res 2001;15:391–4.
21. Wolfsheimer KJ, Peterson ME. Erythrocyte insulin receptors in dogs with spontaneous hyperadrenocorticism. Am J Vet Res 1991;52:917–21.
22. Sukegawa I, Hizuka N, Takano K, et al. Characterization of insulin-like growth factor I receptors on Madin-Darby canine kidney (MDCK) cell line. Endocrinol Jpn 1987;34:339–46.
23. Rave K, Potocka E, Boss AH, et al. Pharmacokinetics and linear exposure of AFRESA compared with the subcutaneous injection of regular human insulin. Diabetes Obes Metab 2009;11:715–20.
24. Plum A, Agerso H, Andersen L. Pharmacokinetics of the rapid-acting insulin analog, insulin aspart, in rats, dogs, and pigs, and pharmacodynamics of insulin aspart in pigs. Drug Metab Dispos 2000;28:155–60.
25. Gilor C, Keel T, Attermeier KJ, et al. Hyperinsulinemic-euglycemic clamps using insulin detemir and insulin glargine in healthy cats [abstract]. J Vet Intern Med 2008;22(3):729.

26. Siebenhofer A, Plank J, Berghold A, et al. Short acting insulin analogues versus regular human insulin in patients with diabetes mellitus. Cochrane Database Syst Rev 2006;(2):CD003287.
27. Mannucci E, Monami M, Marchionni N. Short-acting insulin analogues vs. regular human insulin in type 2 diabetes: a meta-analysis. Diabetes Obes Metab 2009; 11:53–9.
28. Brunner GA, Hirschberger S, Sendlhofer G, et al. Postprandial administration of the insulin analogue insulin aspart in patients with Type 1 diabetes mellitus. Diabet Med 2000;17:371–5.
29. Sears KW, Drobatz KJ, Hess RS. Use of lispro insulin for treatment of dogs with diabetic ketoacidosis [abstract]. J Vet Intern Med 2009;23(3):696.
30. Horvath K, Bock G, Regittnig W, et al. Insulin glulisine, insulin lispro, and regular human insulin show comparable end-organ metabolic effects: an exploratory study. Diabetes Obes Metab 2008;10:484–91.
31. Matsuo Y, Shimoda S, Sakakida M, et al. Strict glycemic control in diabetic dogs with closed-loop intraperitoneal insulin infusion algorithm designed for an artificial endocrine pancreas. J Artif Organs 2003;6:55–63.
32. Appleton DJ, Rand JS, Sunvold GD. Insulin sensitivity decreases with obesity, and lean cats with low insulin sensitivity are at greatest risk of glucose intolerance with weight gain. J Feline Med Surg 2001;3:211–28.
33. Mori A, Sako T, Lee P, et al. Comparison of three commercially available prescription diet regimens on short-term post-prandial serum glucose and insulin concentrations in healthy cats. Vet Res Commun 2009;33:669–80.
34. Heise T, Pieber TR. Towards peakless, reproducible and long-acting insulins. An assessment of the basal analogues based on isoglycaemic clamp studies. Diabetes Obes Metab 2007;9:648–59.
35. Danne T, Datz N, Endahl L, et al. Insulin detemir is characterized by a more reproducible pharmacokinetic profile than insulin glargine in children and adolescents with type 1 diabetes: results from a randomized, double-blind, controlled trial. Pediatr Diabetes 2008;9:554–60.
36. Fakhoury W, Lockhart I, Kotchie RW, et al. Indirect comparison of once daily insulin detemir and glargine in reducing weight gain and hypoglycaemic episodes when administered in addition to conventional oral anti-diabetic therapy in patients with type-2 diabetes. Pharmacology 2008;82:156–63.
37. Monami M, Marchionni N, Mannucci E. Long-acting insulin analogues versus NPH human insulin in type 2 diabetes: a meta-analysis. Diabetes Res Clin Pract 2008;81:184–9.
38. Mori A, Sako T, Lee P, et al. Comparison of time-action profiles of insulin glargine and NPH insulin in normal and diabetic dogs. Vet Res Commun 2008;32:563–73.
39. Marshall RD, Rand JS, Morton JM. Treatment of newly diagnosed diabetic cats with glargine insulin improves glycaemic control and results in higher probability of remission than protamine zinc and lente insulins. J Feline Med Surg 2009;11: 683–91.
40. Roomp K, Rand J. Intensive blood glucose control is safe and effective in diabetic cats using home monitoring and treatment with glargine. J Feline Med Surg 2009;11:668–82.
41. Bennett N, Greco DS, Peterson ME, et al. Comparison of a low carbohydrate-low fiber diet and a moderate carbohydrate-high fiber diet in the management of feline diabetes mellitus. J Feline Med Surg 2006;8:73–84.
42. Weaver KE, Rozanski EA, Mahony OM, et al. Use of glargine and lente insulins in cats with diabetes mellitus. J Vet Intern Med 2006;20:234–8.

43. Hall TD, Mahony O, Rozanski EA, et al. Effects of diet on glucose control in cats with diabetes mellitus treated with twice daily insulin glargine. J Feline Med Surg 2009;11:125–30.

44. Soran H, Younis N. Insulin detemir: a new basal insulin analogue. Diabetes Obes Metab 2006;8:26–30.

45. Hordern SV, Russell-Jones DL. Insulin detemir,does a new century bring a better basal insulin? Int J Clin Pract 2005;59:730–9.

46. Ellmerer M, Hamilton-Wessler M, Kim SP, et al. Mechanism of action in dogs of slow-acting insulin analog O346. J Clin Endocrinol Metab 2003;88: 2256–62.

47. Jonassen I, Havelund S, Ribel U, et al. Biochemical and physiological properties of a novel series of long-acting insulin analogs obtained by acylation with cholic acid derivatives. Pharm Res 2006;23:49–55.

48. Shojaee-Moradie F, Eckey H, Jackson NC, et al. Novel hepatoselective insulin analogues: studies with covalently linked thyroxyl–insulin complexes. Diabet Med 1998;15:928–36.

49. Shojaee-Moradie F, Powrie JK, Sundermann E, et al. Novel hepatoselective insulin analog: studies with a covalently linked thyroxyl-insulin complex in humans. Diabetes Care 2000;23:1124–9.

50. Marshall RD, Rand JS, Morton JM. Glargine and protamine zinc insulin have a longer duration of action and result in lower mean daily glucose concentrations than lente insulin in healthy cats. J Vet Pharmacol Ther 2008;31:205–12.

51. Gilor C, Ridge TK, Attemeier KJ, et al. Pharmacodynamics of insulin detemir and insulin glargine assessed using an isoglycemic clamp method in healthy cats. Am J Vet Res; in press.

52. Roomp K, Rand JS. Evaluation of detemir in diabetic cats managed with a protocol for intensive blood glucose control [abstract]. J Vet Intern Med 2009;23(3):697.

Insulin Resistance in Dogs

Rebecka S. Hess, DVM

KEYWORDS

- Diabetes • Insulin resistance • Dogs • Insulin therapy
- Blood glucose

Resistance to insulin can be divided into two different types. One type of insulin resistance is characterized mainly by inadequate function of endogenous insulin. This form of insulin resistance is important mostly in dogs that are not overtly diabetic and do not require permanent exogenous insulin administration.

The other form of insulin resistance occurs in overtly diabetic dogs when exogenously administered insulin does not have its expected effect. In dogs, this is the most important form of insulin resistance, and therefore it will be discussed first.

DEFINITION OF RESISTANCE TO EXOGENOUS INSULIN

Definitions of resistance to exogenously administered insulin vary, but all are based on the dose of insulin administered and the resultant blood glucose concentrations. Such insulin resistance is suspected when hyperglycemia is present in the face of insulin doses greater than 1.0 to 1.5 U/kg per injection.[1–3]

The degree of hyperglycemia that should raise concern about insulin resistance is also somewhat arbitrary. Hyperglycemia is determined based on serial measurements of blood glucose concentrations, measured every 2 hours over a period of 10 to 12 hours. Hyperglycemia warranting a suspicion for insulin resistance cannot be determined based on a single elevated blood glucose measurement. This is illustrated in **Figs. 1** and **2**. In both graphs, blood glucose concentrations are plotted over a 10-hour period, and food and insulin are given at time zero. **Fig. 1** depicts serial blood glucose measurements in a well-regulated diabetic dog that is clinically normal and is receiving neutral protamine Hagedorn (NPH) insulin at a dose of less than 1.0 U/kg per injection. This dog has high blood glucose concentrations (approaching 400 mg/dL) within 1 hour of eating and receiving insulin, but the blood glucose concentrations are otherwise well within the desired range, and the dog does not have insulin resistance. **Fig. 2** depicts serial blood glucose concentrations in a dog receiving NPH insulin at a dose of 1.0 U/kg per injection. While the maximum blood glucose concentration in both graphs is similar, only the dog in **Fig. 2** is suspected

Department of Clinical Studies–Philadelphia, School of Veterinary Medicine, University of Pennsylvania, 3900 Delancey Street, Philadelphia, PA 19104 6010, USA
E-mail address: rhess@vet.upenn.edu

Vet Clin Small Anim 40 (2010) 309–316
doi:10.1016/j.cvsm.2009.12.001
0195-5616/10/$ – see front matter © 2010 Elsevier Inc. All rights reserved.

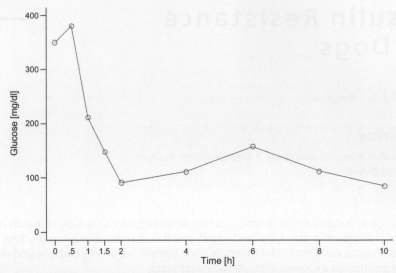

Fig. 1. Serial blood glucose measurements plotted against time. The dog received insulin (<1.0 U/kg per injection) and was fed at time zero. This dog is not insulin resistant even though initial blood glucose concentrations are high.

of having insulin resistance because it has consistently elevated blood glucose concentrations. Therefore, a reasonable definition of insulin resistance is the presence of blood glucose concentrations that are persistently above 200 mg/dL when measured every 2 hours over a 10- to 12-hour period in a diabetic dog receiving an insulin dose greater than 1.0 U/kg.

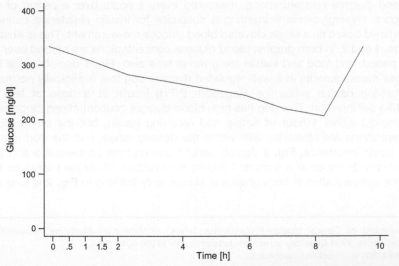

Fig. 2. Serial blood glucose measurements plotted against time. The dog received insulin (1.0 U/kg per injection) and was fed at time zero. This dog has insulin resistance because it has serially elevated blood glucose concentrations.

Another method for defining insulin resistance has recently been described.[1] In this method, the insulin-induced percent of blood glucose suppression is calculated as illustrated in **Fig. 3**. A blood glucose curve is plotted, and the area of interest is defined as the rectangular region between two parallel lines drawn through the value of a blood glucose concentration of 50 mg/dL and through the point of maximum blood glucose concentration (just above 360 mg/dL in the example provided in **Fig. 3**). The vertical lines of each rectangle are drawn through time zero (the time of insulin administration and feeding) and 10 hours later. The area above the blood glucose curve (in light gray in **Fig. 3**), divided by the entire area of the rectangle was defined as the percent of insulin-induced suppression of blood glucose concentration. The mean percent of insulin-induced blood glucose suppression in well-regulated diabetic dogs is 50 ± 17% (median 46%; range 29%–78%). Because the percent suppression and percent resistance add up to 100% in each dog, the percent resistance in well-regulated diabetic dogs is also about 50%.[1] While this method has not been validated in poorly regulated diabetic dogs, it is expected that, with insulin resistance, the percent resistance would be higher.

DIFFERENTIAL DIAGNOSES FOR RESISTANCE TO EXOGENOUSLY ADMINISTERED INSULIN

The reasons for resistance to exogenously administered insulin can be divided into two categories. One category includes causes that result in perceived, but not true, resistance to exogenous insulin. The other category includes conditions that lead to true insulin resistance.

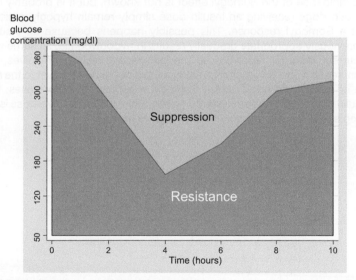

Fig. 3. A blood glucose curve plotted for each dog. The area of interest is defined as the rectangular region between two parallel lines drawn through the value of a blood glucose concentration of 50 mg/dL and through the point of maximal blood glucose concentration (just above 360 mg/dL for this dog). The vertical lines of each rectangle are drawn through time zero (the time of insulin administration and feeding) and 10 hours later. The area above the blood glucose curve (light gray), divided by the entire area of the rectangle is defined as the insulin-induced percent suppression of blood glucose concentration.

Perceived Resistance to Exogenous Insulin

Causes of perceived resistance to exogenous insulin include improper handling of insulin (eg, vigorous shaking of the insulin vial), improper administration of insulin (eg, administration of air instead of insulin or administration of insulin onto the fur instead of into the subcutaneous tissue), or use of the wrong insulin syringe (eg, use of a U-100 syringe with a U-40 insulin product, such as purified porcine insulin zinc suspension [Vetsulin] or human recombinant protamine zinc insulin [ProZinc]). Outdated insulin may also lead to a misperception of insulin resistance and should be suspected in hyperglycemic dogs in which the same insulin vial has been used for longer than 3 months.[3]

The Somogyi effect may also cause the misperception of insulin resistance. The Somogyi effect occurs when pronounced hyperglycemia develops as a response to severe insulin-induced hypoglycemia (*continuous line*, **Fig. 4**). When sudden, severe insulin-induced hypoglycemia develops, protective mechanisms involving secretion of catecholamines (epinephrine and norepinephrine), glucocorticoids, glucagon, and growth hormone result in pronounced hyperglycemia. If the hypoglycemia that preceded the hyperglycemia is not noted, one may mistakenly think that the animal has insulin resistance, when in fact it is very sensitive to insulin, as evidenced by the hypoglycemia. Misinterpretation of the Somogyi effect may result in a potentially fatal outcome, which illustrates the need for a glucose curve. In **Fig. 4**, if blood glucose concentrations in the dog exhibiting the Somogyi effect (*continuous line*) had been measured only 4 to 12 hours after feeding and insulin administration, one could have mistakenly thought that the dog needed a higher dose of insulin. An increase in the insulin dose in this instance could lead to fatal hypoglycemia.

The true incidence of the Somogyi effect is not known, but it is probably not high. Many diabetic dogs receiving an insulin dose simply remain hypoglycemic and do not mount a Somogyi response. This possibly happens because an insulin dose that was previously appropriate gradually results in hypoglycemia, as some unknown mild concurrent disorder resolves. As the concurrent disorder resolves, there is a gradual increase in insulin sensitivity that gives the dog time to adjust to the relatively high dose of insulin and not mount a Somogyi response. In other cases, in which a large insulin overdose was administered erroneously, the insulin overdose is so large that the dog seems unable to mount a Somogyi response.

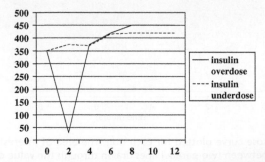

Fig. 4. High blood glucose concentration at 4 to 12 hours after insulin administration and feeding may be seen following insulin-induced hypoglycemia due to insulin overdose (*continuous line,* the Somogyi effect) or when the insulin dose is not high enough (*dashed line*).

Resistance to Exogenous Insulin Due to Concurrent Disease

Many concurrent diseases can cause resistance to exogenous insulin by triggering the secretion of the stress-related, counterregulatory, diabetogenic hormones glucagon, glucocorticoids, catecholamines, and growth hormone. A study of 48 diabetic dogs demonstrated significant linear relationships between serum ketone concentration and concentrations of serum glucagon, cortisol, and norepinephrine, suggesting that poor glycemic regulation (evidenced by high ketone concentrations) may be due to an increase in the concentration of counterregulatory hormones.[4] Treatment of these concurrent disorders generally results in improved glycemic regulation requiring a smaller dose of insulin. However, resolution of these disorders often does not reverse the diabetic state.

Some concurrent disorders also cause insulin resistance because of their specific pathophysiology. For example, increased secretion of glucocorticoids in hyperadrenocorticism, catecholamines in pheochromocytoma, and growth hormone in acromegaly results in insulin resistance regardless of the stress associated with the disease.

The most common concurrent disorders diagnosed in 221 diabetic dogs (including well-regulated and poorly regulated dogs) were hyperadrenocorticism (diagnosed in 23% of dogs), urinary tract infection (21%), acute pancreatitis (13%), neoplasia (5%), and hypothyroidism (4%).[5] In a different study of 127 dogs with diabetic ketoacidosis, in which glycemic regulation was poor, the most common concurrent disorders were acute pancreatitis (diagnosed in 41% of dogs), urinary tract infection (20%), and hyperadrenocorticism (15%).[6]

Some of these conditions, such as neoplasia or hyperadrenocorticism, probably develop simply because the diabetic dog is middle-aged to older and therefore is at increased risk for these concurrent disorders. Other concurrent disorders, such as urinary tract infection or acute pancreatitis, develop specifically because the animal is diabetic.

Diabetic dogs are at increased risk for urinary tract infections because neutrophil adherence to antigens is decreased when serum glucose concentration is increased.[7] Dilute urine and presence of glucose, an excellent substrate for bacterial growth, also increase the risk of urinary tract infections. Other infections, such as pyoderma and pneumonia, have also been associated with insulin resistance in dogs.[5]

It has been suggested that the hypercholesterolemia associated with diabetes mellitus increases the risk of acute pancreatitis in diabetic dogs.[8] Hypothyroidism and diabetes mellitus may develop in the same dog because both are thought to involve immune-mediated destruction of the endocrine gland. It is possible that, in some dogs, this immune-mediated destruction involves both endocrine glands.

Diestrus, pregnancy, or exogenous progesterone administration are all associated with an increase in circulating progesterone concentration. In dogs with acromegaly, progesterone induces growth hormone production in the mammary glands, and, because growth hormone is one of the four counterregulatory or diabetogenic hormones, this results in insulin resistance.[9] Neutering or discontinuation of progesterone administration may lead to resolution of diabetes in some of these dogs.[10]

Other drugs, in addition to progesterone, can cause insulin resistance.[11] Glucocorticoids increase the blood glucose concentration, primarily by increasing hepatic gluconeogenesis and decreasing use of peripheral glucose. Cyclosporin A suppresses insulin secretion in canine pancreatic islet cell cultures and is associated with beta-cell destruction, characterized by degranulation and vacuolization, cytoplasmic swelling, and apoptosis.[12]

The association between anti-insulin antibodies (AIA) and insulin resistance is controversial. A recent study of 220 diabetic dogs treated with insulin extracted from bovine or porcine pancreata found that there was no significant difference in AIA when comparing porcine insulin–treated dogs to control dogs.[13] However, dogs treated with bovine insulin had significantly higher AIA compared to control dogs. Nevertheless, presence of AIA was not associated with the insulin dose or with fructosamine concentration. Therefore, the clinical significance of AIA is not known.[13]

DIAGNOSTIC EVALUATION OF RESISTANCE TO EXOGENOUS INSULIN

When resistance to exogenously administered insulin is encountered, the diagnostic evaluation is determined according to the clinical signs exhibited. For example, if the only clinical signs are polyuria and polydipsia, a urinary tract infection may be suspected, and a sterile urine sample may be submitted for an aerobic culture. Because poorly regulated diabetics often have polyuria and polydipsia due to osmotic diuresis driven by glucosuria, a urine culture is often performed in these dogs, whether or not they have clinical signs traditionally associated with a lower urinary tract infection (such as pollakiuria, hematuria, or dysuria).

If the predominant clinical signs at the time insulin resistance is encountered are vomiting and abdominal pain, then an upper urinary tract infection may still be possible, but acute pancreatitis, should be considered.

Hyperadrenocorticism is a common concurrent disorder in diabetic dogs, and warrants special consideration. The diagnosis of concurrent canine hyperadrenocorticism and diabetes can be challenging because the diseases have similar clinical signs, physical examination findings, and clinicopathologic changes (**Table 1**). Such cases can be complicated because treatment of one disease influences the treatment of the other.

When patients with concurrent diabetes and hyperadrenocorticism are presented, the task of distinguishing one disease from the other may be difficult because of their similar clinical signs and biochemical findings (see **Table 1**). In some cases, the presence of both diseases may be suspected at the onset of clinical signs; in others, suspicion of concurrent hyperadrenocorticism may develop when insulin resistance is encountered during the treatment of diabetes. Regardless of whether concurrent hyperadrenocorticism is suspected initially, it is recommended to treat the diabetes first and diagnose the hyperadrenocorticism later. This recommendation is made for two reasons. First, clinical and clinicopathologic changes suggestive of hyperadrenocorticism will resolve with the treatment of diabetes if they are the result of diabetes only. If the clinical suspicion of hyperadrenocorticism is eliminated after the diabetes is regulated, diagnostic tests for hyperadrenocorticism are unnecessary because clinical signs have resolved. Second, increased secretion of glucocorticoids from stress or illness (eg, unregulated diabetes) can cause false-positive results for hyperadrenocorticism. Adrenal function testing is not recommended in poorly regulated diabetic patients because of the possibility of falsely positive adrenal axis test results due to the secretion of glucocorticoids triggered by the stress of unregulated diabetes.

If treatment with reasonable doses of insulin (up to 1.0–1.5 U/kg) does not lead to resolution of hyperglycemia and clinical signs, then adrenal axis testing is recommended.

If the clinical signs associated with insulin resistance are vague, it may be helpful to evaluate the diabetic patient for the most common concurrent disorders diagnosed in diabetic dogs.

Table 1
Clinical signs, physical examination findings, and clinicopathology in dogs with diabetes mellitus or hyperadrenocorticism

Signalment	Diabetes Mellitus	Hyperadrenocorticism
Breed predisposition	Australian terrier, Samoyed, pug, miniature and toy poodle, miniature schnauzer	Many
Age	Middle-aged to older	Middle-aged to older
Clinical signs		
Polyuria and polydipsia	Yes	Yes
Polyphagia	Yes	Yes
Body condition	Variable	Truncal obesity; muscle wasting of the extremities
Signs of lower urinary tract infection	Possible	Possible
Progression of clinical signs	Usually slow and chronic	Usually slow and chronic
Physical examination		
Hepatomegaly	Yes	Yes
Concurrent infections (pyoderma, pneumonia)	Possible	Possible
Bilateral, symmetric, nonpruritic alopecia	No	Possible
Panting	No	Possible
Cataracts	Possible	No
Complete blood count		
Mature or left-shift neutrophilia	Possible	Possible
Mild polycythemia	Possible	Possible
Thrombocytosis	Possible	Possible
Chemistry screen		
Hyperglycemia	Yes	Possible
Elevated serum alanine aminotransferase	Possible	Possible
Elevated alkaline phosphatase	Possible	Possible
Elevated serum cholesterol and lipemia	Possible	Possible
Urinalysis		
Specific gravity	Variable	Dilute
Glucosuria	Yes	Possible
Urine sediment	May have less than adequate number of leukocytes in response to infection	May have less than adequate number of leukocytes in response to infection

TREATMENT

Treatment of insulin resistance should target the concurrent disease that has been diagnosed. Treatment will therefore vary according to which concurrent disease has been identified. However, regardless of the treatment for the specific concurrent disorder that has been diagnosed, one must be mindful of adjusting the insulin dose appropriately.

When treatment against a concurrent disorder is administered (eg, if trilostane is given to treat pituitary-dependent hyperadrenocorticism), the insulin dose must be decreased to achieve a target blood glucose concentration between 200 and 400 mg/dL. This is because treatment of the concurrent disorder will increase insulin sensitivity. Therefore, a dose of insulin that was ineffective prior to treatment of hyperadrenocorticism could result in good glycemic control after treatment.

REFERENCES

1. Palm C, Boston R, Refsal K, et al. An investigation of the action of NPH human analogue insulin in dogs with naturally-occurring diabetes mellitus. J Vet Intern Med 2009;23:50–5.
2. Feldman EC, Nelson RW. Canine diabetes mellitus. In: Feldman EC, Nelson RW, editors. Canine and feline endocrinology and reproduction. 3rd edition. Philadelphia: WB Saunders; 2004. p. 486–538.
3. Bangstad H-J, Danne T, Deeb LC, et al. ISPAD clinical practice consensus guidelines 2009 compendium. insulin treatment in children and adolescents with diabetes. Pediatr Diabetes 2009;10(Suppl 12):82–99.
4. Durocher LL, Hinchcliff KW, DiBartola SP, et al. Acid-base and hormonal abnormalities in dogs with naturally occurring diabetes mellitus. J Am Vet Med Assoc 2008;232:1310–20.
5. Hess RS, Saunders HM, Thomas J, et al. Concurrent disorders in dogs with diabetes mellitus: 221 cases (1993–1998). J Am Vet Med Assoc 2000;217:1166–73.
6. Hume DZ, Drobatz KJ, Hess RS. Outcome of dogs with diabetic ketoacidosis: 127 dogs (1993–2003). J Vet Intern Med 2006;20:547–55.
7. Latimer KS, Mahaffey EA. Neutrophil adherence and movement in poorly and well-controlled diabetic dogs. Am J Vet Res 1984;45(8):1498–500.
8. Hess RS, Kass P, Shofer F, et al. Evaluation of risk factors for fatal acute pancreatitis in dogs. J Am Vet Med Assoc 1999;214:46–51.
9. Bhatti SFM, Duchateau L, Okkens AC, et al. Treatment of growth hormone excess in dogs with the progesterone receptor antagonist aglepristone. Theriogenology 2006;66(4):797–803.
10. Norman EJ, Wolsky KJ, MacKay GA. Pregnancy-related diabetes mellitus in two dogs. N Z Vet J 2006;54(6):360–4.
11. Murray S, Gasser A, Hess R. Transient hyperglycaemia in a pre-diabetic dog treated with prednisone and cyclosporine A. Aust Vet J 2009;87(9):352–5.
12. Dracheberg CB, Klassen DK, Weir MR, et al. Islet cell damage associated with tacrolimus and cyclosporine: morphological features in pancreas allograft biopsies and clinical correlation. Transplantation 1999;68:396–402.
13. Davison LJ, Walding B, Herrtage ME, et al. Anti-insulin antibodies in diabetic dogs before and after treatment with different insulin preparations. J Vet Intern Med 2008;22:1317–25.

Diabetic Emergencies in Small Animals

Mauria A. O'Brien, DVM

KEYWORDS

- Hyperglycemia • Hyperosmolality • Ketones • Insulin
- Glucagon • Counterregulatory

Diabetic ketoacidosis (DKA) and hyperglycemic hyperosmolar syndrome (HHS) are two interrelated complications of diabetes mellitus. The pathophysiology and treatment for both syndromes is similar but the finer points are discussed in more detail. These conditions can be considered as two ends of a continuous spectrum of decompensated diabetes.[1] More than one third of human cases show significant overlap between DKA and HHS.[2] The definition for each entity varies slightly depending on what reference is consulted, but the basic definition of DKA includes a diagnosis of hyperglycemia, glucosuria, ketonemia, or ketonuria with a metabolic acidosis (pH <7.3, bicarbonate <15 mmol/L).[3,4] HHS is defined as profound hyperglycemia (>600 mg/dL), hyperosmolality (>320 mOsm/kg), pH >7.3, but without significant or detectable ketonemia or ketonuria.[5] HHS was previously referred to as "hyperosmolar nonketotic coma" and "hyperglycemic hyperosmolar nonketotic state," but this definition has expanded to include mild-to-moderate ketonemia, and coma is a rare finding.[4,6] Inherent to these syndromes are significant fluid, electrolyte, and acid-base disturbances.[7] In most cases there is a coexisting or confounding disease process that can substantially affect prognosis. A recent study showed that the two most important factors predicting mortality in human DKA were severe concurrent illness and pH less than 7.[8]

PATHOPHYSIOLOGY

Key to the pathogenesis of DKA and HHS is a relative deficiency of insulin. Insulin is produced and secreted by pancreatic beta cells in response to a rise in blood glucose concentrations.[9] Insulin stimulates cellular uptake of glucose to provide energy for most cells of the body, particularly muscle, adipose tissue, and hepatic cells. When insulin is deficient, hyperglycemia develops by three processes: (1) increased gluconeogenesis, (2) accelerated glycogenolysis, and (3) impaired glucose use by tissues.[6] Despite elevated serum glucose concentrations with insulinopenia, the body's cells become "starved" for energy. When glucose is unavailable as a substrate, most cells

Department of Veterinary Clinical Medicine, University of Illinois at Urbana-Champaign, 1008 West Hazelwood Drive, Urbana, IL 61802, USA
E-mail address: maobrien@illinois.edu

Vet Clin Small Anim 40 (2010) 317–333
doi:10.1016/j.cvsm.2009.10.003
0195-5616/10/$ – see front matter © 2010 Elsevier Inc. All rights reserved.

are able to use free fatty acids (FFAs) as an energy source. Certain cells and organs have absolute requirements for glucose; these include the brain, retina, and germinal epithelium of the gonads.[7] Brain cells are unique in that they do not require insulin for glucose uptake,[9] but unlike most tissues, the brain cannot use fatty acids for energy. Instead, ketone bodies can provide the brain with two thirds of its energy needs in periods of fasting or starvation.[10]

Insulin hinders lipolysis through the inhibition of hormone-sensitive lipase. Hormone-sensitive lipase is an enzyme responsible for the hydrolysis of triglycerides into fatty acids. Lipolysis generates and liberates FFAs into the circulation.[9] FFAs are taken up by hepatocytes and converted predominantly to triglycerides and, to a lesser degree, into ketones. Uncomplicated diabetics convert most of the excess FFA to triglycerides and ketone production is low enough as to be manageable by the body (**Fig. 1**).[7]

What distinguishes DKA from uncomplicated diabetes mellitus is the relative lack of insulin combined with an increase in counterregulatory hormones. Glucagon, cortisol, epinephrine, and growth hormone comprise the counterregulatory hormones, and the presence of a secondary or coexisting disease process is believed to result in

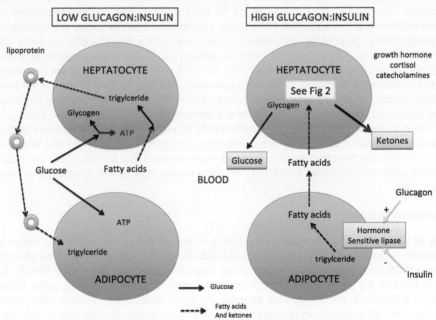

Fig. 1. Ratio of glucagon/insulin determines the use and storage of glucose and fatty acids by hepatocytes and adipocytes. When insulin concentrations are high (*left panel*), glucose is converted to energy (ATP) in most cells and is stored as glycogen in hepatocytes. Fatty acids are converted to triglycerides in hepatocytes. From the hepatocyte the triglycerides are transported by lipoproteins for storage in adipocytes. When insulin concentrations are low, as in DKA (*right panel*), the glycogen is liberated as glucose from the hepatocyte. Hormone-sensitive lipase, stimulated by glucagon and inhibited by insulin, transforms the triglycerides in adipocytes to free fatty acids. Under the stimulus of glucagon and other counter-regulatory hormones, free fatty acids are oxidized to ketones. (*Adapted from* Laffel L. Ketone bodies: a review of physiology, pathophysiology and application of monitoring in diabetes. Diabetes Metab Res Rev 1999;15:412–25; with permission.)

increased concentrations of these "stress" hormones.[11] Indeed, DKA is characterized by an increased glucagon/insulin ratio.[7] This elevated ratio leads to a state of enhanced gluconeogenesis by inhibition and stimulation of certain enzymes of the glycolysis pathway.[6] A recent study in dogs revealed that the glucagon/insulin ratio is more important than the individual hormone concentrations, and that ketonemia and ketoacidosis can be controlled without the need to regulate serum glucose concentrations. Many diabetic dogs in this study had normal concentration of insulin but ketone formation still occurred.[12] A study of dogs with DKA demonstrated insulin concentrations that ranged from less than the concentrations seen in uncomplicated diabetics to normal concentrations.[13] This supports the theory that many DKA events may be precipitated by a period of "relative" insulin resistance, potentially brought about by a secondary disease process.

Counterregulatory Hormones

Glucagon is the predominant hormone implicated in the pathogenesis of DKA and HHS. Pancreatic alpha cells secrete glucagon in response to low blood glucose concentrations, and its actions oppose those of insulin. Glucagon increases gluconeogenesis and promotes glycogenolysis. Glucagon also activates adipose cell lipase, which increases the concentration of FFA and inhibits storage of triglycerides in the liver.[9] With the relative or absolute lack of insulin in DKA, cellular demand for glucose stimulates the release of glucagon. Because of a complex second messenger cascade system, a small amount of glucagon leads to large quantities of glucose being produced.[7,9] Even when hepatic stores are depleted of glycogen, glucagon accelerates gluconeogenesis and increases the extraction rate of amino acids from the circulation to act as available substrates for the process.[9] As a result of glucagon's effects, glucose concentrations increase and, without insulin present, lead to hyperglycemia. A vicious cycle ensues and glucose concentrations continue to rise.

Glucagon also promotes ketogenesis by shifting hepatocyte production of triglycerides to the production of FFA. Normally, insulin inhibits the production of FFA by stimulation of malonyl coenzyme A (CoA). Malonyl CoA inhibits fatty acid oxidation. In the absence of insulin, malonyl CoA activity is low and glucagon stimulates FFA uptake into the mitochondria by increasing hepatic levels of carnitine. Carnitine is a carrier protein used by the enzyme carnitine palmitoyltransferase I, which shuttles FFAs into the mitochondria. From this point the FFAs can either enter the citric acid cycle or be converted into ketone bodies (acetoacetic acid and β-hydroxybutyric acid). In DKA, the citric acid cycle becomes overwhelmed because of insufficient substrates and ketogenesis proceeds. As ketone concentrations rise the body becomes unable to metabolize them efficiently and hyperketonemia results (**Fig. 2**).[10]

In addition to glucagon, other counterregulatory hormones (epinephrine, cortisol, growth hormone) are secreted and contribute to the pathogenesis of DKA and HHS. Together these hormones contribute to hyperglycemia and ketonemia by promoting lipolysis and stimulating gluconeogenesis and glycogenolysis. Cortisol increases protein catabolism, providing amino acid precursors for gluconeogenesis.[4] Cortisol and epinephrine stimulate hormone-sensitive lipase, which is normally inhibited by insulin. Hormone-sensitive lipase mediates the breakdown of triglycerides to glycerol and FFAs in adipose tissue.[4] Glycerol is a precursor for gluconeogenesis in the liver and kidney, whereas FFAs are oxidized to ketones in hepatic mitochondria. Ketonemia is minimally or not present in HHS probably because there is sufficient insulin to limit lipolysis but it is insufficient to counter hyperglycemia.[6] Another hypothesis is that the absence of ketones may be caused by lower concentrations of FFAs, increased portal vein insulin concentrations, or both.[14]

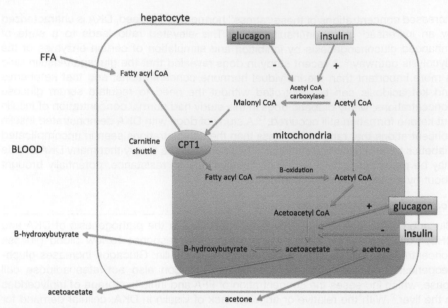

Fig. 2. Free fatty acids (FFA) are transported into hepatic mitochondria by the carnitine shuttle, driven by carnitine palmitoyltransferase 1 (CPT1). Acetyl-CoA carboxylase catalyzes the production of malonyl CoA from acetyl CoA. Because malonyl CoA inhibits CPT1, decreased activity of acetyl-CoA carboxylase stimulates transport of fatty acids into the mitochondria. Glucagon inhibits acetyl-CoA carboxylase and stimulates the conversion of acetoacetyl CoA into acetoacetate. Acetoacetate is reduced to β-hydroxybutyrate and acetone is formed by spontaneous decarboxylation of acetoacetate. (*Adapted from* Laffel L. Ketone bodies: a review of physiology, pathophysiology and application of monitoring in diabetes. Diabetes Metab Res Rev 1999;15:412–25; with permission.)

Secondary or concurrent diseases contribute to the severity of DKA or HHS. It is believed that the increase in counterregulatory hormone concentrations is likely because of coexisting disease. In human patients, the two most common precipitating factors are inadequate insulin dosing and infection.[2,4,6,14] Poorly regulated diabetics are at increased risk of infection because of impaired neutrophil adhesion, chemotaxis, phagocytosis,[15,16] and bactericidal activity.[16,17] In veterinary patients, acute pancreatitis, urinary tract infection, hyperadrenocorticism, neoplasia, pneumonia, pyelonephritis, and chronic renal disease[17] have all been reported concurrently with DKA or HHS.[18–21]

Recent studies have shown that hyperglycemic states are proinflammatory and produce reactive oxygen species.[2,22–24] Intensive insulin therapy is said to exert an anti-inflammatory effect because proinflammatory markers return to normal with the initiation of insulin therapy.[25] Intensive insulin therapy is being used in critically ill nondiabetic patients who are hyperglycemic on presentation or become hyperglycemic after presentation. Tightly regulating blood glucose concentrations between 80 and 120 mg/dL has shown a significant improvement in mortality in critically ill patients.[26,27]

Electrolyte and Acid-base Disturbances

The combined effects of hyperglycemia, ketonemia, and a comorbid process can lead to significant electrolyte derangements in DKA and HHS. Glucosuria and ketonemia-induced osmotic diuresis result in severe fluid losses through intercellular fluid movement and renal losses. In DKA, urinary ketoanion excretion is less than that of glucose. Excretion of ketoanions obligates urinary cation excretion as sodium, potassium, and ammonium salts, which contributes to the solute diuresis.[6] Hyponatremia also results from the effects of hyperglycemia as free water shifts from the intracellular to the extracellular compartment causing a dilution of plasma sodium.[14] This effect can be accounted for by the following rule: for every 100 mg/dL increase in serum glucose there is a decrease in serum sodium (by dilution) of 1.6 mmol/L.[28] Insulin deficiency can also contribute to solute loss because insulin stimulates salt and water reabsorption in the proximal and distal tubules and phosphate reabsorption in the proximal tubule.[6]

Significant hypokalemia is present in many cases of DKA. It is common for patients to present with normal to slightly elevated serum potassium concentrations, but most animals with DKA have severe total body depletion of potassium.[14] The acidosis of DKA leads to displacement of potassium from intracellular stores to the extracellular space in exchange for hydrogen ions, but potassium concentrations are affected by multiple causes.[28,29] Volume depletion, from lack of intake combined with vomiting, diarrhea, and osmotic diuresis, causes secondary hyperaldosteronism, which promotes urinary potassium excretion.[30] The osmotic diuresis caused by the glucosuria and ketonuria leads to fluid shifts from the intracellular to the extracellular compartment upsetting the balance between intracellular and extracellular potassium, and this leads to potassium movement out of the cell. Intercompartmental potassium shifts can vary depending on the type of acidosis (mineral vs organic); by tissue type; and by the pH of body fluids.[29] Decreased dietary intake of potassium, and loss through vomiting, exacerbates whole-body potassium depletion. Renal dysfunction, by promoting hyperglycemia and reducing urinary potassium excretion, also contributes to potassium balance.[31] In addition, insulin deficiency promotes intracellular proteolysis, further impairing potassium entry into the cells. Plasma potassium concentrations increase in the face of whole-body potassium depletion.[4] Magnesium, calcium, and phosphorus are also depleted in DKA, mostly by excess renal excretion.[14]

Fluid loss is multifactorial in DKA and HHS. The osmotic diuresis secondary to glycosuria and ketonuria leads to significant fluid loss. Coexisting disease processes, decreased fluid intake, and fluid loss through diarrhea or vomiting also contribute.[11] Patients with HHS reportedly have more extensive fluid losses than those with DKA. Under normal conditions, the kidneys excrete excess glucose above a certain threshold and prevent further hyperglycemia. The more chronic disease state of HHS causes decreased intravascular volume leading to decreases in glomerular filtration rate (GFR) and plasma glucose concentrations rise. Combined with chronic renal disease, common in many HHS patients, there is more water loss than sodium loss, and hyperosmolality results.[5]

DKA is characterized as a metabolic acidosis, specifically an elevated anion gap metabolic acidosis. The overproduction of the ketoacids, β-hydroxybutyrate and acetoacetate, is the main contributor to the acidosis. Both dissociate completely at physiologic pH resulting in the production of hydrogen ions and ketoanions. The rapid accumulation of hydrogen ions saturates the bicarbonate buffering system and metabolic acidosis develops.[10,11] The cause of the metabolic acidosis in this case is the accumulation of ketoanions, reflected by an increased anion gap.[28,32] Hypovolemia, brought about by significant fluid losses, causes lactic acidosis and contributes to the metabolic acidosis. The third ketone body, acetone, is formed by spontaneous decarboxylation of acetoacetate. Although it is present in high concentrations in

DKA it does not contribute to the acidosis because, unlike the other two ketones, it does not dissociate. Acetone is slowly excreted by the lungs and generates the distinctive, "sweet" smelling breath of patients with DKA.[10] Because of the slow excretion it takes longer to correct ketonemia than hyperglycemia.[14,33]

Patients with HHS have severe hyperglycemia with plasma glucose concentrations often above 600 mg/dL. This reflects the more severe dehydration seen with this syndrome. The osmotic diuresis combined with lack of fluid intake and loss through vomiting leads to hypovolemia and decreased GFR. Severe hyperglycemia can only occur with reduced GFR because most glucose entering the kidney in excess of the renal threshold should be excreted in the urine.[34] The profound hyperglycemia then exacerbates the osmotic diuresis.[28] Human patients with HHS tend to be older, type 2 diabetics with concurrent diseases, such as chronic kidney disease or congestive heart failure.[5,35] A retrospective study by Koenig and coworkers[17] found similar concurrent disease processes in cats, although this study did not include any cats with ketosis. The definition of HHS is changing and now includes conditions of mild or moderate ketosis. HHS has also been referred to as "hyperosmolar nonketotic coma," which is a misnomer because coma is an inconsistent finding in humans[6,36] and animals with the disorder.[34]

CLINICAL FEATURES
History and Physical Examination

Patients with DKA or HHS are either currently being treated for diabetes mellitus; are newly diagnosed diabetics; or have historical signs of polyuria, polydipsia, and weight loss. Most dogs and cats are middle-aged to older with no gender predilection.[37] In the acute phase before presentation, usually 1 to 3 days, owners typically report partial or complete anorexia, often with vomiting or diarrhea.[38] Cats may also exhibit signs of weakness or gait change.[39] Lethargy and a dull, unkempt hair coat are often present. Very few dogs and cats are presented with altered mentation or decreased consciousness,[38] although cats with HHS were more likely to have neurologic signs than cats with DKA in one study.[17] Patients with severe metabolic acidosis may display Kussmaul respirations (slow, deep breathing),[37] which can be misinterpreted as respiratory distress. DKA may develop more acutely than HHS.[4] There are very few veterinary reports of HHS, but a study in cats showed no difference in the time of onset of clinical signs between HHS and DKA cats, but cats with HHS had been diagnosed with diabetes for a longer period of time before presentation.[17] Humans with HHS have a more insidious onset of clinical signs,[4] making the clinical outcome worse.

Diagnostics

All patients suspected of having DKA or HHS should have a thorough work-up. This includes a complete blood count, serum chemistry panel, serum electrolytes, blood gas panel, urinalysis, urine culture, abdominal ultrasound, and thoracic radiographs. Many of the diagnostics tests are aimed at investigation of comorbid conditions.

Complete blood count may show an elevated hematocrit secondary to dehydration.[7] Anemia may be present and is more common in cats because of the susceptibility to Heinz body formation and red blood cell oxidative injury.[40] In one study, 50% of dogs had nonregenerative anemia, left shift neutrophilia, and thrombocytosis.[18,41] Leukocytosis is a more common finding in humans[2,14] and cats.[19,42]

In dogs, serum chemistry analysis panel can show elevated alanine aminotransferase, aspartate aminotransferase, and alkaline phosphatase. Hypovolemia, causing decreased hepatic perfusion and hepatocellular damage, can lead to increased serum liver enzyme activity.[7] Increased transaminase activity can also be seen in cats, especially those with concurrent hepatic lipidosis.[38] Increased alkaline phosphatase activity, hypertriglyceridemia, and hypercholesterolemia are common in dogs with hypercortisolism or pancreatitis. Because most dogs and cats with DKA and HHS are severely dehydrated, azotemia is a common finding. High blood-urea-nitrogen and creatinine concentrations may be caused by renal or prerenal causes.[7] Hyperglycemia is found in all diabetics, but patients with HHS have serum glucose concentrations above 600 mg/dL.

Electrolyte abnormalities can include hyponatremia, hypochloremia, hypocalcemia, and hypomagnesemia. Hyponatremia can be secondary to hypertriglyeridemia. (pseudohyponatremia)[43] or secondary to significant hyperglycemia causing fluid shifts from the intracellular compartment and dilution of the sodium.[38] Increased, decreased, or normal concentrations of potassium and phosphorus can be seen. Acid-base findings in DKA include metabolic acidosis (pH <7.35, Hco_3 <15 mEq/L) with compensatory respiratory alkalosis and increased anion gap. Acid-base status in patients with HHS can be normal.[5]

Hyperglycemia alters serum osmolality.[17,44,45] The severity of hyperosmolality can be variable in DKA but patients with HHS have hyperosmolar serum by definition. Osmolality is measured by an osmometer that uses the freezing point of a solution to estimate the amount of osmotically active particles. Measurement of osmolality is superior to calculating osmolality because of the ability to measure volatile substances in a solution.[46] Unfortunately, it may not be practical for a veterinary practice to have an osmometer on hand. Several equations have been devised to calculate osmolality to better approximate the measured value. The most commonly used calculation (also referred to as "total calculated osmolality" [Osm_T]) is:

Extracellular fluid osmolality (mOsm/kg) = $2(Na^+ + K^+)$ + Glucose/18 + BUN/2.8

A recent publication showed this equation to be best at approximating the measured Osm_T.[46] Published normal calculated osmolality values range from 290 to 310 mOsm/kg.[47-49] The effective osmolality (Osm_E)[50] is another frequently used equation:

$Osm_E = 2(Na^+)$ + Glucose/18[50]

Sodium and glucose are the two solutes that contribute the most to serum tonicity and urea is considered an ineffective osmole given its ability to diffuse across membranes. Hypertonicity results from an increase in the concentration of solutes that do not cross the cell membrane. Hyperosmolality is defined as effective serum osmolality above 320 mOsm/kg in humans[5] and above 330 mOsm/kg in cats[45] and dogs.[44] A study of cats with HHS found the median Osm_T was 384 mOsm/kg and median Osm_E was 344.1 mOsm/kg.[17] With an increase in the tonicity of the extracellular fluid, cellular dehydration results as water shifts from the intracellular compartment to the extracellular compartment. This is most significant in brain cells. Neurologic signs (disorientation, ataxia, lethargy, seizures, and coma) develop with worsening cellular dehydration. In defense against this, cells create intracellular solutes called "idiogenic osmoles" that help to diminish the osmotic movement of water out of the cell. Serum ketone concentrations are not routinely measured in DKA but are known to contribute to the osmolality. Measurement of the osmole gap (measured Osm_T, calculated Osm_T) produces a mean osmolar gap of 29 mOsm/kg. This gap has been shown to decrease to insignificant values within 24 hours of therapy for DKA.[51–53] Because ketoanions are presumed to fully dissociate at physiologic pH they are not considered to contribute significantly to tonicity but based on the osmolar gap do contribute to osmolality.[53,54] It has been thought that the higher the osmolality the worse the neurologic signs or risk of cerebral edema,[55] but this subject is still unresolved.[56–58] Recent studies in children and adults relate severe acidemia with the most significant neurologic signs.[30,59] A veterinary study of dogs with DKA showed a relationship between acidosis and outcome but did not specifically correlate pH with neurologic signs.[18]

Historically, measurement of ketones has been through the nitroprusside reaction on urine reagent strips. These strips only measure acetoacetate and acetone but 75% to 90% of ketone bodies are made up of β-hydroxybutyrate and acetoacetate.[53,54] β-hydroxybutyrate is formed from acetoacetate in the presence of hydrogen ions; the more acidotic is an animal, the more β-hydroxybutyrate is formed. Some patients are significantly dehydrated and urine sample cannot be obtained initially. The limitations of the urine strips prompted the development of assays to detect β-hydroxybutyrate in blood. These assays are considered reliable for diagnosing and monitoring response to therapy in people and can be used as an alternative to the urine ketone test.[60,61] Commercially available hand-held meters have been validated in dogs and cats.[62–64] Heparinized plasma can also be tested using a urine dipstick, and this accurately reflects acetoacetate and acetone concentrations in diabetic dogs and cats.[65]

Serum lactate concentrations have been found to be high in dogs and cats with diabetes. This may be secondary to severe dehydration and decreased perfusion, or may be caused by decreased metabolism of lactate.[12] Lactic acidosis may contribute to the overall metabolic state,[11] although the blood lactate did not correlate with venous pH in several studies.[12,17,18,66]

Urinalysis is positive for glucose and may be positive for ketones. Because of the limitations of the nitroprusside reagent in the urine sticks, ketones may be negative initially, and subsequently positive as β-hydroxybutyrate is converted to acetoacetate. Care should be taken to look for signs of urinary tract infection. Bacterial culture and antibiotic sensitivity testing should be done regardless of the urinary white cell count because 20% of dogs with DKA have positive growth on aerobic culture of the urine despite the lack of pyuria.[18]

MANAGEMENT

Successful treatment of DKA or HHS is complex and involves the correction of many derangements. The goals of treatment encompass (1) restoring intravascular volume, (2) correcting dehydration, (3) correcting electrolyte disturbances, (4) correcting acid-base imbalance, (5) decreasing blood glucose concentrations, (6) ridding the body of detectable ketones, and (7) treating any underlying or coexisting disease.

Ideally, most patients with DKA and HHS should be hospitalized in a 24-hour facility equipped with the ability to perform basic biochemical and electrolyte testing in-house. A peripheral IV catheter should be placed to allow for IV fluid therapy. Many patients are significantly hypovolemic and require initial stabilization with IV fluid boluses. Perfusion parameters (heart rate, pulse quality, mentation, mucous membrane color, capillary refill time, blood pressure) should dictate whether fluid boluses are necessary before rehydration rates are instituted. Insulin should never be started in a hypovolemic animal because it can cause a fluid shift from the extracellular to the intracellular compartment, worsening the already depleted intravascular volume.[5]

Most commercially available crystalloid solutions are adequate for resuscitation and rehydration. Traditionally, the fluid of choice is 0.9% sodium chloride because many patients are hyponatremic (uncorrected) on presentation.[2,4,14,67–70] Saline (0.9%) is a nonbuffered solution and is known to cause a temporary, hyperchloremic metabolic acidosis when infused intravenously.[14,71,72] This type of acidosis results from a loss of bicarbonate rather than a gain of organic acid.[28] Buffered crystalloid solutions (eg, lactated Ringers, Normosol-R, Plasma-lyte) have the benefit of an adequate sodium content with the advantage of a buffer (lactate, acetate, gluconate) to aid in the resolution of the metabolic acidosis.[41] Close monitoring of perfusion, hydration status, and electrolytes is the most important aspect of treatment regardless of the type of crystalloid chosen. Fluid therapy alone contributes significantly to the initial decrease in glucose, ketones, and counterregulatory hormones by increasing the GFR and urinary excretion.[28]

Most patients should be rehydrated for at least several hours before instituting insulin therapy. Fluid deficits are calculated based on estimations of dehydration:

% dehydration $\times$ body weight (kg) $\times$ 1000 mL/kg = mL of fluid deficit

These estimates are subjective and should be reassessed often in the early stages of therapy. Rehydration is typically performed over a relatively short period of time (6–24 hours), although the speed of replacement should depend on the individual patient's hemodynamic, cardiovascular, osmotic, and neurologic status. Recall that many patients are hyperglycemic and ketonemic for hours to days and this contributes to continued osmotic diuresis and must continually be accounted for when determining or adjusting fluid rates.

Rehydration of the HHS patient often requires more conservative fluid therapy. Because of the severe dehydration and hyperosmolality, rehydration should occur more slowly than in DKA to minimize sudden changes in glucose or sodium concentrations, which affect the Osm_E. Rapid changes in Osm_E could lead to sudden shifting of fluid to the intracellular compartment, which could lead to cerebral edema. Children with DKA are more prone to developing cerebral edema in the acute phases of therapy. Different mechanisms have been proposed, but many studies have shown a sudden change in Osm_E has been associated with the occurrence of cerebral edema.[73] Recent recommendations include slower rehydration rates and lower insulin dosing initially to produce a gradual decline in Osm_E as reflected by a decrease in serum glucose and a concomitant increase in serum sodium.[56,74] Severe neurologic signs related to hypertonicity were not reported in a recent study, even in cats with marked hyperglycemia.[44] No neurologic complications were noted in another study in cats with HHS.[17] If neurologic signs are present on presentation, as is more typical with veterinary patients with HHS,[34] treatment should be more conservative: rehydrate over 24 to 48 hours and use a lower insulin dose (**Table 1**). Also, patients with HHS can be minimally ketotic, so insulin is needed more for treating hyperglycemia than for ketonemia. Severely affected patients with altered mentation (obtunded, stuporous, or comatose), abnormal cranial nerve reflexes, or seizures should be treated with mannitol (0.5–1.5 g/kg).[75]

Given that most commercially available isotonic solutions for IV fluid therapy are sodium based, most sodium abnormalities are corrected with standard IV fluid therapy alone. In diabetics, rising serum glucose concentrations lead to an increase in serum osmolality. Fluid shifts intravascularly to compensate, and this leads to a dilutional effect on sodium concentrations. To determine if the degree of hyponatremia is appropriate for the degree of hyperglycemia the following formula should be applied: for every 100 mg/dL increase in glucose there should be a 1.6 mg/dL decrease in sodium.

Table 1
Insulin adjustments with changes in blood glucose concentrations

Blood Glucose (mg/dL)	IV Fluids[a]	Rate of Administration of Insulin Solution (mL/h)[b]
>250	0.9% NaCl	10
200–250	0.45% NaCl + 2.5% dextrose	7
150–200	0.45% NaCl + 2.5% dextrose	5
100–150	0.45% NaCl + 2.5% dextrose	5
<100	0.45% NaCl + 5% dextrose	Stop insulin infusion

50 mL of the solution is run through the IV line before connecting to the patient because insulin binds to plastic.

[a] Lactated ringer's solution (LRS), Normosol-R, Plasmalyte can be substituted for 0.9% NaCl or 0.45% NaCl.

[b] Regular crystalline insulin is added to 250 mL of 0.9% NaCl or LRS at a dose of 2.2 U/kg (dogs) or 1.1 U/kg (cats). This dose can be halved for HHS or hyperosmolar patients.

Data from Macintire DK, Drobatz KJ, Haskins SC, et al. Manual of small animal emergency and critical care medicine. Baltimore: Lippincott Williams and Wilkins; 2005. p. 296–333.

If the corrected sodium is within the normal range, the sodium concentration normalizes as the blood glucose concentration is reduced. If the corrected sodium is low, this indicates sodium wasting has occurred, and a higher sodium solution can be used, at least initially. If the uncorrected sodium level is normal in the face of hyperglycemia this represents an excess of free water loss and hyperosmolality. This is more commonly encountered in patients with HHS. Fluid therapy should be more conservative and hypotonic fluids should be avoided to minimize rapid shifts in osmolality that could lead to cerebral edema.[39]

Potassium balance should be addressed immediately. Although serum concentrations can be normal or elevated on presentation, most patients with DKA or HHS have whole-body potassium depletion. Fluid therapy can cause a shift of potassium intracellularly leading to increased GFR and renal potassium excretion. Hypokalemia causes muscle weakness, cervical ventroflexion (cats), cardiac arrhythmias,[76] and respiratory muscle failure in severely affected animals.[39] Standard veterinary texts[41,69,77] have tables for potassium replacement (**Table 2**). Potassium chloride is

Table 2
Potassium supplementation guidelines

Serum K$^+$ (mEq/L)	KCl Supplementation (mEq/L)	Max Delivery Rate[a] (mL/kg/h)
3.5–5	20	24
3–3.4	30	16
2.5–2.9	40	11
2–2.4	60	8
<2	80	6

Calculating the volume of KCl to give as a bolus infusion:
Total volume of KCl = (Ideal K$^+$ - Patient K$^+$) × Estimated vascular volume#.
#Dogs = 90 mL/kg × body wt (kg); Cats = 60 mL/kg × body wt (kg).
Take the total volume of KCl and dilute with 2–3 times the volume in saline.
Give over 10 minutes while monitoring EKG.
Best given through a central catheter to avoid pain.

[a] Above this rate exceeds 0.5 mEq/kg/h.

Data from Macintire DK, Drobatz KJ, Haskins SC, et al. Manual of small animal emergency and critical care medicine. Baltimore: Lippincott Williams and Wilkins; 2005. p. 296–333.

added to the IV fluid bag based on serum potassium concentrations. Most sources warn against administering more than 0.5 mEq/kg/h, but life-threatening hypokalemia (<2 mEq/L) should be treated using a dose of 0.5 to 0.9 mEq/kg/h[78] for the first hour followed by reassessment. Insulin therapy should be withheld until potassium concentrations are closer to normal (>3.5 mEq/L) because insulin therapy promotes intracellular movement of potassium.

After 4 to 8 hours of fluid therapy, or when the patient is better hydrated, a central venous catheter should be placed. This allows frequent blood sampling without repeated venipuncture. Insulin therapy should be started at this time, and frequent glucose monitoring, with insulin dose adjustment. Insulin is essential in the treatment of DKA; without it ketonemia does not resolve. Insulin lowers ketone body concentrations by three independent mechanisms: (1) insulin lipolysis, thereby lowering FFA availability for ketogenesis; (2) insulin retards ketone body production within the liver; and (3) insulin enhances peripheral ketone body metabolism.[79] Several veterinary texts and references[20,41,69] provide easy-to-follow tables used for determining insulin dosages based on serum glucose concentrations (**Box 1**). Although not necessarily ketotic, patients with HHS also need insulin to reduce hyperglycemia in a controlled manner.

Regular insulin is used initially when treating DKA and HHS. There has been a progression in veterinary medicine to treat patients with insulin as a constant rate infusion (CRI) rather than using the traditional method of intramuscular injections. This is mirrored in human medicine, and a "low-dose" infusion of regular insulin is considered the standard of care for treatment of complicated DKA and HHS.[30,80] Studies show lower mortality rates in human patients treated with intravenous insulin infusions.[4] Intramuscular administration of insulin in veterinary patients should be reserved for uncomplicated cases or in cases in which financial restrictions limit the use of CRIs. Critically ill patients with DKA and HHS are fluid-depleted and must be rehydrated adequately before intramuscular injections of insulin are given. Circulatory compromise may hinder the delivery of insulin to tissues or deliver it an unpredictable manner. This could lead to acute hypoglycemia or sudden osmolality changes that can compromise the patient and complicate recovery. The goal of insulin therapy is to decrease the glucose concentration by no more than 50 to 75 mg/dL/h. If the glucose level drops below 250 to 300 mg/dL and ketones are still present, glucose should be added to the IV fluids (see **Table 1**). Once the patient is hydrated and eating, a longer-acting insulin formulation can be used.[34]

Insulin has other uses besides glycemic control. Anti-inflammatory properties of insulin have been shown in both diabetic and nondiabetic patients with hyperglycemia. One study demonstrated increased circulating concentrations of growth hormone, cortisol, cytokines, and markers of cardiovascular risk, and oxidative stress in lean

---

Box 1
Helpful calculations

1. $Na^+_{Corr} = Na^+_{uncorr} + ([(GLU_{patient} - GLU_{normal})/GLU_{normal}] \times 1.6)$

2. $Osm_T (mOsm/L) = 2(Na^+ + K^+) + (GLU/18) + (BUN/2.8)$

3. $Osm_E (mOsm/L) = 2(Na^+ + K^+) + (GLU/18)$

4. Anion gap = $(Na^+ + K^+) - (Cl^- + Hco_3^-)$

5. Dehydration estimate (mL) = % dehydration $\times$ body wt (kg) $\times$ 1000 mL/kg

and obese ketoacidotic diabetic patients. Concentrations of these substances returned to normal shortly after initiation of insulin therapy. The well-known phenomenon of leukocytosis without obvious infection in humans with hyperglycemic crises may be caused by an increase in proinflammatory mediators.[22] A second study demonstrated increased C-reactive protein concentrations in critically ill patients with hyperglycemia, and normalization with insulin therapy.[25] Studies have demonstrated increased survival in critically ill nondiabetic patients treated with insulin to maintain euglycemia.[26,27] It may not have been euglycemia per se but the anti-inflammatory effect of insulin that led to improved survival in these studies, and further investigation of this phenomenon is needed. In addition to strict monitoring of glucose, sodium, and potassium, phosphorus concentrations should be monitored closely. As with hypokalemia, hypophosphatemia may not be apparent until after insulin therapy has started. Clinical signs of hypophosphatemia include muscle weakness and hemolytic anemia. Phosphorus can be added to IV fluids in the form of potassium phosphate (KPO_4). Dosing ranges from 0.03 to 0.12 mmol/kg/h[41] are added to the IV fluids. Alternatively, one third to one half of the calculated dose of potassium supplementation can be added as KPO_4, with KCl used for the remainder.[39] Potassium phosphate is reportedly incompatible with lactated ringer's solution.[75] The serum phosphorus concentration should be measured 4 to 6 hours after starting fluid therapy and adjusted accordingly. Iatrogenic hyperphosphatemia could lead to secondary hypocalcemia.

Hypomagnesemia is becoming a more recognized and appreciated syndrome in critical illness and DKA. Signs can be clinically inapparent and may manifest themselves through refractory hypokalemia. Magnesium depletion promotes urinary potassium loss[81] and potassium concentrations do not normalize without replacement of magnesium.[76] Magnesium sulfate (4 mEq/mL) is added to the IV fluids and given as a CRI at a dose of 0.5 to 1 mEq/kg/d.[41]

The metabolic acidosis of DKA typically resolves with fluid therapy and insulin alone. Traditionally, sodium bicarbonate was used to treat the acidosis of DKA but this therapy is falling out of favor. The American Diabetes Association does list it as a treatment option for patients with a pH less than 7 after 1 hour of fluid therapy but there are no prospective randomized studies to prove its benefits.[80] Sodium bicarbonate therapy can be dangerous in DKA for several reasons. Like insulin, bicarbonate drives potassium intracellularly potentially worsening hypokalemia. Bicarbonate shifts the oxyhemoglobin curve to the left decreasing oxygen release at the tissue level,[80] and can lead to paradoxic central nervous system acidosis, fluid overload, lactic acidosis, persistent ketosis,[4] and cerebral edema.[82,83]

COMPLICATIONS

Complications encountered in treatment of DKA or HHS can be prevented by diligent monitoring. Unfortunately, repeated blood sampling can lead to anemia and the need for blood transfusions. Cats, having eight reactive sulfhydryl groups on each hemoglobin tetramer, are prone to Heinz body anemia in critical illness. There is some evidence to suggest that ketosis can exacerbate this condition.[40] Acute hemolytic anemia can also occur if extracellular phosphorus concentrations drop precipitously with insulin therapy. Serum phosphorus concentrations below 1.5 mg/dL are associated with risk for hemolysis.

Overzealous insulin administration can lead to hypoglycemia, although this is easily remedied by discontinuing the insulin CRI. If ketones are still present, insulin administration should be reinstated to stop ketogenesis, and dextrose supplementation of the IV fluids may be needed (see **Table 1**).

An uncommon complication, seen in children with DKA but rarely in veterinary medicine, is cerebral edema after initiation of therapy. Cerebral edema occurs in roughly 1% of children with DKA and is associated with a mortality rate of 40% to 90%.[84] Pathophysiologic mechanisms for this complication remain controversial. Ischemia and reperfusion injury, inflammation,[24] increased blood flow, intracellular osmolyte generation, osmotic "imbalance," and cytotoxins have all been implicated.[56] Proposed contributing factors includes high initial plasma glucose concentrations, excessive IV fluid administration, and persistent hyponatremia despite resolution of hyperglycemia.[58] Hypocapnia, low pH, hyperkalemia, increased blood-urea-nitrogen/creatinine ratio, and sodium bicarbonate use have been associated with increased risk.[84–86] Cerebral edema in DKA is usually noted within 12 to 24 hours of initiating therapy, and some have suggested that cerebral edema may be present before therapy is started. Two schools of thought are present among clinicians. Some believe in the cytotoxic theory, which holds that osmotic gradients are created by overzealous fluid and insulin therapy. The second theory, the vasogenic theory, proposes a disruption of vascular permeability in the blood-brain barrier is the major mechanism behind cerebral edema in DKA.[87] Regardless, the most recent recommendations include more conservative fluid and insulin therapy initially to minimize rapid drops in the effective osmolality.[56,58,74,87,88]

PROGNOSIS

Prognosis in DKA and HHS is largely dependent on the concurrent disease process. Previous retrospective veterinary studies have listed mortality rates ranging from 26% to 30%[18–20] for DKA and 65% for HHS.[17] Although mortality rates are lower, there is a worse prognosis with HHS compared with DKA in human patients (10%–50% vs 1.9%–10%, respectively).[5,6,80] Regardless of species, without resolution of comorbid processes, the outcome of DKA or HHS worsens. In the study of cats with HHS there was only a 12% long-term survival rate, with most of the cats dying in hospital.[17] The complicated pathogenesis of DKA and HHS creates a considerable medical challenge for the veterinary practitioner. Clients and clinicians should be prepared for the financial, emotional, and unpredictable outcome of these diabetic complications.

REFERENCES

1. Bhowmick SK, Levens KL, Rettig KR. Further thoughts on hyperosmolar hyperglycemic crisis. Endocr Pract 2006;12(4):477–8.
2. Kitabchi AE, Nyenwe EA. Hyperglycemic crises in diabetes mellitus: diabetic ketoacidosis and hyperglycemic hyperosmolar state. Endocrinol Metab Clin North Am 2006;35(4):725–51, viii.
3. Feldman EC, Nelson RW. Diabetic ketoacidosis. In: Feldman EC, Nelson RW, editors. Canine and feline endocrinology and reproduction. 3rd edition. St. Louis (MO): Saunders; 2004. p. 580–615.
4. English P, Williams G. Hyperglycaemic crises and lactic acidosis in diabetes mellitus. Postgrad Med J 2004;80(943):253–61.
5. Stoner GD. Hyperosmolar hyperglycemic state. Am Fam Physician 2005;71(9): 1723–30.
6. Kitabchi AE, Umpierrez GE, Murphy MB, et al. Management of hyperglycemic crises in patients with diabetes. Diabetes Care 2001;24(1):131–53.
7. Kerl ME. Diabetic ketoacidosis: pathophysiology and clinical laboratory presentation. Compendium 2001;23(3):220–8.

8. Efstathiou SP, Tsiakou AG, Tsioulos DI, et al. A mortality prediction model in diabetic ketoacidosis. Clin Endocrinol 2002;57:595–601.
9. Guyton AC. Insulin, glucagon, diabetes mellitus. In: Guyton AC, Hall JE, editors. Textbook of medical physiology. 10th edition. Philadelphia: W.B. Saunders; 2000. p. 884–98.
10. Laffel L. Ketone bodies: a review of physiology, pathophysiology and application of monitoring in diabetes. Diabetes Metab Res Rev 1999;15:412–25.
11. Boysen SR. Fluid and electrolyte therapy in endocrine disorders: diabetes mellitus and hypoadrenocorticism. Vet Clin North Am Small Anim Pract 2008;38(3): 699–717, xiii–xiv.
12. Durocher LL, Hinchcliff KW, DiBartola SP, et al. Acid-base and hormonal abnormalities in dogs with naturally occurring diabetes mellitus. J Am Vet Med Assoc 2008;232(9):1310–20.
13. Parsons SE, Drobatz KJ, Lamb SV, et al. Endogenous serum insulin concentration in dogs with diabetic ketoacidosis. J Vet Emerg Crit Care 2002;12(3):147–52.
14. Chiasson JL, Aris-Jilwan N, Belanger R, et al. Diagnosis and treatment of diabetic ketoacidosis and the hyperglycemic hyperosmolar state. CMAJ 2003;168(7): 859–66.
15. Alexiewicz JM, Kumar D, Smogorzewski M, et al. Polymorphonuclear leukocytes in non-insulin-dependent diabetes mellitus: abnormalities in metabolism and function. Ann Intern Med 1995;123(12):919–24.
16. Repine JE, Clawson CC, Goetz FC. Bactericial function of neutrophils from patients with acute bacterial infections and from diabetics. J Infect Dis 1980; 142(6):869–75.
17. Koenig A, Drobatz KJ, Beale AB, et al. Hypergylcemic, hyperosmolar syndrome in feline diabetics: 17 cases (1995–2001). J Vet Emerg Crit Care 2004;14(1):30–40.
18. Hume DZ, Drobatz KJ, Hess RS. Outcome of dogs with diabetic ketoacidosis: 127 dogs (1993–2003). J Vet Intern Med 2006;20(3):547–55.
19. Bruskiewicz KA, Nelson RW, Feldman EC, et al. Diabetic ketosis and ketoacidosis in cats: 42 cases (1980–1995). J Am Vet Med Assoc 1997;211(2):188–92.
20. Macintire DK. Treatment of diabetic ketoacidosis in dogs by continuous low-dose intravenous infusion of insulin. J Am Vet Med Assoc 1993;202(8):1266–72.
21. Nichols R, Crenshaw KL. Complications and concurrent disease associated with diabetic ketoacidosis and other severe forms of diabetes mellitus. Vet Clin North Am Small Anim Pract 1995;25(3):617–24.
22. Stentz FB, Umpierrez GE, Cuervo R, et al. Proinflammatory cytokines, markers of cardiovascular risks, oxidative stress, and lipid peroxidation in patients with hyperglycemic crises. Diabetes 2004;53:2079–86.
23. Kitabchi AE, Stentz FB, Umpierrez GE. Diabetic ketoacidosis induces in vivo activation of human T-lymphocytes. Biochem Biophys Res Commun 2004;315:404–7.
24. Hoffman WH, Stamatovic SM, Andjelkovic AV. Inflammatory mediators and blood brain barrier disruption in fatal brain edema of diabetic ketoacidosis. Brain Res 2009;1254:138–48.
25. Hansen TK, Thiel S, Wouters PJ, et al. Intensive insulin therapy exerts anti-inflammatory effects in critically ill patients and counteracts the adverse effect of low mannose-binding lectin levels. J Clin Endocrinol Metab 2003;88:1082–8.
26. Van den Berghe G, Wouters PJ, Weekers F, et al. Intensive insulin therapy in the critically ill patients. N Engl J Med 2001;19:1359–67.
27. Van den Heuvel I, Vanhorebeek I, Van den Berghe G. The importance of strict blood glucose control with insulin therapy in the intensive care unit. Curr Diabet Rev 2008;4:227–33.

28. Kandel G, Aberman A. Selected developments in the understanding of diabetic ketoacidosis. Can Med Assoc J 1983;128:392–7.
29. Adrogue M, Madias NE. Changes in plasma potassium concentration during acute acid-base disturbances. Am J Med 1981;71:456–67.
30. Wolfsdorf J, Glaser N, Sperling MA. Diabetic ketoacidosis in infants, children and adolescents. Diabetes Care 2006;29(5):1150–9.
31. Adrogue HJ, Lederer ED, Suki WN, et al. Determinants of plasma potassium levels in diabetic ketoacidosis. Medicine (Baltimore) 1986;65:163–72.
32. Wellman ML, DiBartola SP, Kohn CW. Applied physiology of body fluids in dogs and cats. In: DiBartola SP, editor. Fluid, electrolyte, and acid-base disorders in small animal practice. 3rd edition. St Louis (MO): Saunders Elsevier; 2006. p. 3–25.
33. De Beer K, Michael S, Thacker M, et al. Diabetic ketoacidosis and hyperglycaemic hyperosmolar syndrome: clinical guidelines. Nurs Crit Care 2008;13(1):5–11.
34. Koenig A. Hyperglycemic hyperosmolar syndrome. In: Silverstein DC, Hopper K, editors. Small animal critical care medicine. St. Louis (MO): Saunders Elsevier; 2009. p. 291–4.
35. MacIsaac RJ, Lee LY, McNeil KJ, et al. Influence of age on the presentation and outcome of acidotic and hyperosmolar diabetic emergencies. Intern Med J 2002; 32(8):379–85.
36. Kitabchi AE, Umpierrez GE, Murphy MB, et al. Hyperglycemic crises in patients with diabetes mellitus. Diabetes Care 2001;24(1):154–61.
37. Nelson RW. Diabetes mellitus. In: Ettinger SJ, Feldman BF, editors, Textbook of veterinary internal medicine, vol. 2. 6th edition. St. Louis (MO): Elsevier Saunders; 2005. p. 1563–91.
38. Schaer M. Diabetic ketoacidosis and hyperglycemic hyperosmolar syndrome. In: Ettinger SJ, Feldman BF, editors, Textbook of veterinary internal medicine, vol. 1. 6th edition. St. Louis (MO): Elsevier Saunders; 2005. p. 424–8.
39. Kerl ME. Diabetic ketoacidosis: treatment recommendations. Compendium 2001; 23(4):330–40.
40. Christopher MM, Broussard JD, Peterson ME. Heinz body formation associated with ketoacidosis in diabetic cats. J Vet Intern Med 1995;9(1):24–31.
41. Hess RS. Diabetic ketoacidosis. In: Silverstein DC, Hopper K, editors. Small animal critical care medicine. St. Louis (MO): Saunders Elsevier; 2009. p. 288–91.
42. Crenshaw KL, Peterson ME. Pretreatment clinical and laboratory evaluation of cats with diabetes mellitus: 104 cases (1992–1994). J Am Vet Med Assoc 1996;209(5):943–9.
43. DiBartola SP. Disorders of sodium and water: hypernatremia and hyponatremia. In: DiBartola SP, editor. Fluid, electrolyte, and acid-base disorders in small animal practice. 3rd edition. St. Louis (MO): Saunders Elsevier; 2006. p. 47–79.
44. Schermerhorn T, Barr SC. Relationships between glucose, sodium and effective osmolality in diabetic dogs and cats. J Vet Emerg Crit Care 2006;16(1):19–24.
45. Kotas S, Gerber L, Moore LE, et al. Changes in serum glucose, sodium, and tonicity in cats treated for diabetic ketosis. J Vet Emerg Crit Care 2008;18(5): 488–95.
46. Barr JWI, Pesillo-Crosby SA. Use of the advanced micro-osmometer model 3300 for determination of a normal osmolality and evaluation of different formulas for calculated osmolarity and osmole gap in adult dogs. J Vet Emerg Crit Care 2008;18(3):270–6.
47. Macintire DK. Emergency therapy of diabetic crises: insulin overdose, diabetic ketoacidosis, and hyperosmolar coma. Vet Clin North Am Small Anim Pract 1995;25(3):639–50.

48. Chew DJ, Leonard M, Muir WW. Effect of sodium biacarbonate infusion on serum osmolality, electrolyte concentrations, and blood gas tensions in cats. Am J Vet Res 1991;52:12.
49. Hardy RM, Osborne CA. Water deprivation test in the dog: maximal normal values. J Am Vet Med Assoc 1979;174:479.
50. Rose BD, Post TW. Clinical physiology of acid-base and electrolyte disorders. 5th edition. New York: McGraw-Hill; 2001.
51. Davidson DF. Excess osmolal gap in diabetic ketoacidosis explained. Clin Chem 1992;38:755–8.
52. Puliyel J, Puliyel M, Hincliffe R. Hypertonicity in diabetic ketoacidosis. Paper presented at: International Symposium on Diabetes, 1997; Chaing Mai Thailand.
53. Puliyel J. Osmotonicity of acetoacetate: possible implications for cerebral edema in diabetic ketoacidosis. Med Sci Monit 2003;9(4):Br130–3.
54. Coppack S. Diabetes mellitus. New York: Churchill-Livingstone; 1995.
55. Fulop M, Rosenblatt A, Kreitzer SM, et al. Hyperosmolar nature of diabetic coma. Diabetes 1975;24(6):594–9.
56. Friedman AL. Choosing the right fluid and electrolytes prescription in diabetic ketoacidosis. J Pediatr 2007;150:455–6.
57. Glaser N, Wooten-Gorges SL, Marcin JP, et al. Mechanisms of cerebral edema in children with diabetic ketoacidosis. J Pediatr 2004;145:164–71.
58. Edge JA, Jakes RW, Roy Y, et al. The UK case-control study of cerebral oedema complicating diabetic ketoacidosis in children. Diabetologia 2006;49:2002–9.
59. Edge JA, Roy Y, Bergomi A, et al. Conscious level in children with diabetic ketoacidosis is related to severity of acidosis and not to blood glucose concentration. Pediatr Diab 2006;7:11–5.
60. Tantiwong P, Puavilai G, Ongphiphadhanakul B, et al. Capillary blood beta-hydroxy butyrate measurement by reagent strip in diagnosing diabetic ketoacidosis. Clin Lab Sci 2005;18(3):139–44.
61. Harris S, Ng R, Syed H, et al. Near patient blood ketone measurements and their utility in predicting diabetic ketoacidosis. Diabet Med 2004;22:221–4.
62. Di Tommaso M, Aste G, Rocconi F, et al. Evaluation of a portable meter to measure ketonemia and comparison with ketonuria for diagnosis of canine diabetic ketoacidosis. J Vet Intern Med 2009;23(3):466–71.
63. Hoenig M, Dorfman M, Koenig A. Use of a hand-held meter for the measurement of blood beta-hydroxybutyrate in dogs and cats. J Vet Emerg Crit Care 2008;18(1):86–7.
64. Duarte R, Simoes DM, Franchini ML, et al. Accuracy of serum beta-hydroxybutyrate measurements for the diagnosis of diabetic ketoacidosis in 116 dogs. J Vet Intern Med 2002;16(4):411–7.
65. Brady MA, Dennis JS, Wagner-Mann C. Evaluating the use of plasma hematocrit samples to detect ketones utilizing urine dipstick colorimetric methodology in diabetic dogs and cats. J Vet Emerg Crit Care 2003;13(1):1–6.
66. Christopher MM, Broussard JD, Fallin CW, et al. Increased serum D-lactate associated with diabetic ketoacidosis. Metabolism 1995;44(3):287–90.
67. Kitabchi AE, Umpierrez GE, Fisher JN, et al. Thirty years of personal experience in hyperglycemic crises: diabetic ketoacidosis and hyperglycemic hyperosmolar state. J Clin Endocrinol Metab 2008;93(5):1541–52.
68. Hardern RD, Quinn ND. Emergency management of diabetic ketoacidosis in adults. Emerg Med J 2003;20:210–3.
69. Panciera DL. Fluid therapy in endocrine and metabolic disorders. In: DiBartola SP, editor. Fluid, electrolyte, and acid-base disorders in small animal practice. 3rd edition. St. Louis (MO): Saunders Elsevier; 2006. p. 478–89.

70. Macintire DK, Drobatz KJ, Haskins SC, et al. Manual of small animal emergency and critical care medicine. Baltimore (MD): Lippincott Williams and Wilkins; 2005. p. 296–333.
71. Morris CG, Low J. Metabolic acidosis in the critically ill: part 2. Causes and treatment. Anaesthesia 2008;63:396–411.
72. Handy JM, Soni N. Physiological effects of hyperchloraemia and acidosis. Br J Anaesth 2008;101(2):141–50.
73. Rother KI, Schwenk WF. Effect of rehydration fluid with 75 mmol/L of sodium on serum sodium concentration and serum osmolality in young patients with diabetic ketoacidosis. Mayo Clin Proc 1994;69:1149–53.
74. Hoorn EJ, Carlotti AP, Costa LAA, et al. Preventing a drop in effective plasma osmolality to minimize the likelihood of cerebral edema during treatment of children with diabetic ketoacidosis. J Pediatr 2007;150:467–73.
75. Plumb DC. Veterinary drug handbook. 5th edition. Ames (IA): Blackwell; 2005.
76. Marino PL. Potassium. The ICU book. 2nd edition. Baltimore (MD): Williams and Wilkins; 1998. p. 647–59.
77. Nichols R, Crenshaw KL. Complications and concurrent disease associated with diabetic ketoacidosis and other severe forms of diabetes mellitus. In: Bonagura JD, editor. Current veterinary therapy XII. Philadelphia: W.B. Saunders; 1995. p. 384–7.
78. Hamill RJ, Robinson LM, Wexler HR, et al. Efficacy and safety of potassium infusion therapy in hypokalemic critically ill patients. Crit Care Med 1991;19(5): 694–9.
79. Keller U, Lustenberger M, Muller-Brand J, et al. Human ketone body production and utilization studied using tracer techniques: regulation by free fatty acids, insulin, catecholamines, and thyroid hormones. Diabet/Metab Rev 1989;5(3): 285–98.
80. Kitabchi AE, Umpierrez GE, Murphy MB, et al. Hyperglycemic crises in adult patients with diabetes. Diabetes Care 2006;29(12):2739–48.
81. Whang R, Flink EB, Dyckner T, et al. Magnesium depletion as a cause of refractory potassium depletion. Arch Intern Med 1985;145:1686–9.
82. Green SM, Rothrock SG, Ho JD, et al. Failure of adjunctive bicarbonate to improve outcome in severe pediatric diabetic ketoacidosis. Ann Emerg Med 1998;31:41–8.
83. Aschner JL, Poland RL. Sodium bicarbonate: basically useless therapy. Pediatrics 2008;122(4):831–5.
84. Glaser N, Barnett P, McCaslin I, et al. Risk factors for cerebral edema in children with diabetic ketoacidosis. N Engl J Med 2001;344(4):264–9.
85. Dunger DB, Sperling MA, Acerini CL, et al. ESPE/LWPES consensus statement on diabetic ketoacidosis in children and adolescents. Arch Dis Child 2004;89: 188–94.
86. Edge JA, Hawkins MM, Winter DL, et al. The risk and outcome of cerebral oedema developing during diabetic ketoacidosis. Arch Dis Child. 2001;85:16–22.
87. Sperling MA. Cerebral edema in diabetic ketoacidosis: an underestimated complication? Pediatr Diab 2006;7:73–4.
88. Fiordalisi I, Novotny WE, Holbert D, et al. An 18-yr prospective study of pediatric diabetic ketoacidosis: an approach to minimizing the risk of brain herniation during treatment. Pediatr Diab 2007;8:142–9.

Endocrine Hypertension in Small Animals

Claudia E. Reusch, DVM*, Stefan Schellenberg, DVM,
Monique Wenger, DVM

KEYWORDS

- Hypertension • Hyperaldosteronism • Hypercortisolism
- Pheochromocytoma • Hyperthyroidism • Diabetes mellitus

In human medicine, systemic hypertension has long been recognized as a major medical and public health issue, especially with regard to cardiovascular disease. In the most recent report of the Joint National Committee on Prevention, Detection, Evaluation, and Treatment of High Blood Pressure, hypertension was defined as systolic/diastolic blood pressure greater than or equal to 140/90 mm Hg. Systolic/diastolic pressures less than 120/80 mm Hg are considered normal, and blood pressures between the two values have been allocated to the newly introduced category of prehypertension.[1] For decades, physicians have considered diastolic pressure more important than systolic pressure. It has recently become clear, however, that hypertension-associated risks are more accurately attributed to systolic pressure, which is now the primary focus of treatment regimens.[2]

In dogs and cats, the importance of hypertension was first recognized approximately 15 to 20 years ago. Guidelines similar to those established for humans have recently been developed and published as the Consensus Statement of the American College of Veterinary Internal Medicine (ACVIM).[3] There is some controversy with regard to the threshold value at which individual animals are considered hypertensive. This primarily reflects differences between the various studies on blood pressure measurements in healthy dogs and cats and recognition of substantial interbreed differences in dogs.[3,4] Although studies have not determined if a change in systolic or diastolic pressure is more damaging, there has been an emphasis on addressing systolic hypertension in dogs and cats. Currently, blood pressure in pets is classified into four categories according to risk of tissue injury (**Table 1**). As blood pressure rises, there is progressive risk of damage to the so-called end organs or target organs, such as brain, heart, kidney, and eye. The most common adverse effects, which include

Clinic for Small Animal Internal Medicine, Vetsuisse Faculty, University of Zurich, Winterthurerstrasse 260, 8057 Zurich, Switzerland
* Corresponding author.
E-mail address: creusch@vetclinics.uzh.ch (C.E. Reusch).

Vet Clin Small Anim 40 (2010) 335–352
doi:10.1016/j.cvsm.2009.10.005
0195-5616/10/$ – see front matter © 2010 Elsevier Inc. All rights reserved.

Table 1
Classification of blood pressure in dogs and cats based on risk for future target-organ damage, according to the American College of Veterinary Internal Medicine Consensus Statement

Risk Category	Systolic Blood Pressure (mm Hg)	Diastolic Blood Pressure (mm Hg)	Risk of End-Organ Damage
I	<150	<95	Minimal
II	150–159	95–99	Mild
III	160–179	100–119	Moderate
IV	≥180	>120	Severe

Data from Brown S, Atkins C, Bagley R, et al. Guidelines for the identification, evaluation, and management of systemic hypertension in dogs and cats. J Vet Intern Med 2007;21:542–58.

hypertensive retinopathy, intraocular hemorrhage, and hypertensive encephalopathy, are seen when the systolic blood pressure exceeds 180 mm Hg, particularly when the increase is acute. Organ damage, especially damage involving the kidneys, has also been reported with systolic blood pressures less than 180 mm Hg. The threshold for tissue injury is not known, however, and is assumed to be approximately 160 mm Hg in cats and most breeds of dogs (**Table 2**).[5]

Table 2
Target-organ damage due to hypertension, adapted from the American College of Veterinary Internal Medicine Consensus Statement

Tissue	Hypertensive Injury	Clinical Findings Indicative of Target-Organ Damage
Kidney	Progression of chronic kidney disease	Serial increases in creatinine, or decrease in glomerular filtration rate, proteinuria, microalbuminuria
Eye	Retinopathy/choroidopathy	Acute onset blindness Exudative retinal detachment Retinal hemorrhage/edema Retinal vessel tortuosity or perivascular edema Papilledema Vitreal hemorrhage Hyphema Secondary glaucoma Retinal degeneration
Brain	Encephalopathy Stroke	Centrally localizing neurologic signs (eg, lethargy, seizures, acute onset of altered mention, altered behavior, disorientation, balance disturbances)
Heart and vessels	Left ventricular hypertrophy Cardiac failure	Left ventricular hypertrophy Gallop rhythm Arrhythmias Systolic murmur Evidence of cardiac failure Hemorrhage (eg, epistaxis, stroke)

Data from Brown S, Atkins C, Bagley R, et al. Guidelines for the identification, evaluation, and management of systemic hypertension in dogs and cats. J Vet Intern Med 2007;21:542–58.

Hypertension is classified as idiopathic (primary or essential) or secondary. In animals with idiopathic hypertension, persistently elevated blood pressure is not caused by an identifiable underlying or predisposing disease. Until recently, more than 95% of cases of hypertension in humans were diagnosed as idiopathic. New studies have shown, however, a much higher prevalence of secondary causes, such as primary hyperaldosteronism.[6–8] Primary hypertension is thought to be rare in dogs.[5] For cats, the ACVIM Consensus Statement cites two studies in which the prevalence of primary hypertension was approximately 18% to 20%.[9,10] Those results must be interpreted cautiously, however, because subclinical chronic kidney disease and primary hyperaldosteronism may have been overlooked.

Secondary hypertension is elevation in blood pressure because of an underlying identifiable cause. In dogs and cats, secondary hypertension is the most prevalent form and is subclassified into renal and endocrine hypertension. This review focuses on the most common causes of endocrine hypertension in dogs and cats.

BLOOD PRESSURE MEASUREMENT

According to the Consensus Statement of the ACVIM, a leading cause of inaccurate results using indirect measurement devices is technical error associated with personnel inexperience.[3] Therefore, to obtain reliable results, the person making the measurements should be patient and skilled in the handling of animals, clients, and equipment. Blood pressure can be measured indirectly using a noninvasive technique or directly by catheterizing a peripheral artery. The latter method is considered the gold standard; however, it is technically challenging, uncomfortable for patients, and, therefore, not usually feasible in a clinical setting. Most veterinarians rely on indirect methods, which include Doppler flow detection, oscillometry, or the recently introduced high-definition oscillometry.

Regardless of which method is used, it is important to remember that blood pressure is a variable hemodynamic phenomenon that is influenced by many factors. As in people, it is normal for blood pressure to vary throughout the day in cats and dogs. In dogs, blood pressure decreases during sleep or rest and increases significantly during periods of activity.[11,12] In addition to these physiologic fluctuations, stress or anxiety can result in considerable increases in blood pressure. This so-called white-coat effect may lead to a false diagnosis of hypertension.[13] To minimize this effect, animals should not be subjected to any examinations or manipulations before blood pressure has been measured. Instead, patients should be allowed to acclimatize in a quiet room 5 to 10 minutes, and the first blood pressure readings should be discarded. It is noteworthy that in dogs, there may be long-term adaptation to blood pressure measurement. The authors recently showed that repeated measurements over several days resulted in a significant decrease in blood pressure values in dogs (**Fig. 1**). Based on initial measurements, 8 of 12 healthy dogs satisfied conventional criteria for the diagnosis of hypertension. On the second and third evaluations, however, only one dog fulfilled the criteria, and on subsequent evaluations, no dog was considered hypertensive.[14] Rather, blood pressure measurements should be repeated on at least 2 additional days, which is similar to recommendations in human medicine.[15] In addition to stress or anxiety, many other factors are known to affect blood pressure. Cuff size contributes to variations in results because undersized cuffs overestimate blood pressure and oversized cuffs underestimate it. In dogs, a cuff size of approximately 40% of the circumference of the limb is recommended and a value of 30% to 40% is advocated in cats. Cuff location (forelimb, hind limb, or base of the tail) may also alter blood pressure results, especially systolic readings. Therefore,

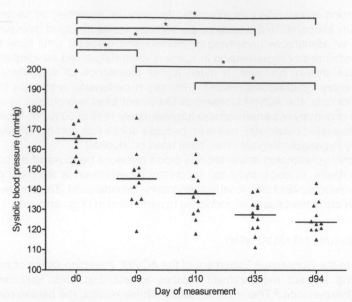

Fig. 1. Systolic blood pressure measurement with a Doppler device in 12 beagle dogs over time (median and individual values are given) *P<.05. (*From* Schellenberg S, Glaus TM, Reusch CE. Effect of long-term adaptation on indirect measurements of systolic blood pressure in conscious untrained beagles. Vet Rec 2007;161:418–21; with permission.)

measurements should always be taken at the same body location for monitoring a patient's blood pressure. In all cases, it is essential to remember that the cuff must be placed at the level of the heart, regardless of the location of the cuff or the position of an animal.

PRIMARY HYPERALDOSTERONISM

The first case of feline primary hyperaldosteronism was described in 1983.[16] Since then, the disease has been diagnosed with increased frequency. Although no data are available concerning the true prevalence, it is assumed that the disease is more common than initially thought. This hypothesis is based on data from human medicine, in which increased disease awareness led to a more systematic screening of the hypertensive population, resulting in a strong increase in prevalence. Only three cases of canine primary hyperaldosteronism have been published to date,[17–19] and three additional cases are described by Feldman and Nelson.[20]

In human medicine, approximately two-thirds of patients have bilateral idiopathic adrenal hyperplasia whereas approximately one-third have aldosterone-producing adenomas (aldosteronomas).[21] Typical findings are systemic hypertension, hypokalemia, and metabolic acidosis. Because screening for the disease is becoming more common and diagnosis is generally being made earlier, however, the prevalence of hypokalemia is decreasing, and currently, the majority of patients are normokalemic at the time of diagnosis.[22,23] Currently, 5% to 10% of the general hypertensive population and 20% of patients with severe or resistant hypertension suffer from primary hyperaldosteronism.[24] The degree of hypertension is usually moderate to severe, and patients with aldosteronoma tend to have higher blood pressure than patients with idiopathic hyperaldosteronism.

The consequences of increased aldosterone concentration are retention of sodium and water in the distal and collecting tubules of the kidneys. This results in increased intravascular volume and increased urinary potassium and hydrogen excretion. Excessive circulating concentrations of aldosterone also induce vasoconstriction and lead to an increase in peripheral vascular resistance. The two central mechanisms responsible for the development of hypertension in primary hyperaldosteronism are expansion of plasma and extracellular fluid volume and increase in total peripheral vascular resistance. Aldosterone itself has proinflammatory and profibrotic properties resulting in vascular, cardiac, and renal lesions. In human patients, this leads to an increased incidence of cardiovascular events, a higher rate of urinary albumin excretion, and higher prevalence of metabolic syndrome in comparison with matched patients suffering from essential hypertension.[25–27] The pathophysiology of aldosterone-associated hypertension in cats is thought to be identical to that in humans.

The majority of cats with primary hyperaldosteronism have been shown to have unilateral carcinomas, whereas adenomas and hyperplasia have been reported less frequently.[16,28–36] Clinical signs include weakness with associated cervical ventroflexion, mydriasis, and blindness because of hypertensive retinopathy; some cats also show polyuria/polydipsia. Almost all cats described to date have been hypokalemic at the time of diagnosis. As in human medicine, however, it is possible that hyperaldosteronism is overlooked in cats with normal serum potassium concentrations. A more systematic screening for primary hyperaldosteronism may improve diagnosis and thus increase the prevalence of the disease. This hypothesis is supported by a recent case report,[34] in which a mass in the region of the right adrenal gland was detected by chance during abdominal ultrasonography in a normokalemic cat presented for pollakiuria. Further evaluation was initially declined by the owner, but 4 months later the cat was diagnosed with primary hyperaldosteronism when it was presented for weakness, cervical ventroflexion, and hypokalemia. Unfortunately, the blood pressure had not been recorded at the initial examination.

Based on data available to date, the prevalence of hypertension in cats with primary hyperaldosteronism seems high. Blood pressure was recorded in 30 cases, 26 of which were hypertensive (**Table 3**).[28–36] The severity ranged from mild to severe (185–270 mm Hg), and the most common sequelae were retinal detachment and ocular bleeding.

Initial treatment should be directed toward alleviation of hypertension and hypokalemia by using an aldosterone antagonist (spironolactone 1 mg/kg every 12 hours orally) and a calcium channel blocker (amlodipine besylate 0.625–1.25 mg/cat every 24 hours orally) and supplementing potassium as needed. Subsequent adrenalectomy is the treatment of choice for animals without tumor metastasis. In the few cases described in the literature and in two cases seen at the authors' hospital, hypertension resolved after surgery. In cases in which adrenalectomy is not feasible (eg, metastasized tumor, bilateral tumor, or hyperplasia), medical treatment with spironolactone and amlodipine besylate should be continued. The two drugs combined seem to lead to resolution of hypertension in most cases.[35]

HYPERADRENOCORTICISM

Hyperadrenocorticism is one of the most common endocrine disorders in dogs but is rare in cats. In approximately 85% of cases, endogenous hyperadrenocorticism is caused by a pituitary tumor, which autonomously secretes adrenocorticotropic hormone, resulting in chronic excess of glucocorticoids. The remaining 15% are caused by primary adrenal hypersecretion of cortisol. The disease has an insidious

Table 3
Data on blood pressure measurements in cats with primary hyperaldosteronism and dogs with hyperadrenocorticism or pheochromocytoma. In some studies, diastolic and mean blood pressure were recorded; however, to facilitate comparison, only systolic blood pressure values are listed.

Endocrinopathy (Species)	No. of Animals Revealing Hypertension (Total No. of Animals with Blood Pressure Measurements)	Measuring Technique	Definition of Systolic Hypertension (mm Hg)	Range of Systolic Blood Pressure (mm Hg) in All Animals	References
Primary aldosteronism (cat)	0 (1)	Indirect, Doppler	Not given	130–140	MacKay et al, 1999[28]
	2 (2)	Indirect, Doppler	>180	230–250	Flood et al, 1999[29]
	0 (1)	Indirect, method not given	Not given	135	Moore et al, 2000[30]
	1 (1)	Indirect, Doppler	>180	190	Rijnberk et al, 2001[31]
	0 (1)	Method not given	Not given	170	DeClue et al, 2005[32]
	11 (12)	Indirect, Doppler	>170	160–250	Ash et al, 2005[35]
	10 (10)	Method not given	>199	185–270	Javadi et al, 2005[36]
	1 (1)	Indirect, Doppler	Not given	200	Rose et al, 2007[33]
	1 (1)	Indirect, method not given	Not given	205	Renschler and Dean, 2009[34]
Hyperadrenocorticism (dog)	31 (36)	Indirect, oscillometric	>160	160–190 (27), >190 (4)	Ortega et al, 1996[51]
	9 (13)	Indirect, Doppler	Not given	>200	Goy-Thollot et al, 2002[52]
	2 (2)	Direct	Not given	>169	Littmann et al, 1988[49]
	8 (12)	Indirect, Doppler	>150	Not given	Novellas et al, 2008[53]
Pheochromocytoma (dog)	1 (1)	Indirect, oscillometric	Not given	200–240	Williams and Hackner, 2001[72]
	0 (1)	Indirect, Doppler	Not given	200–240	Whittemore et al, 2001[73]
	1 (1)	Indirect, Doppler	Not given	110	Brown et al, 2007[3]
	6 (7)	Indirect, Doppler	>160	240	Gilson et al, 1994[69]
	10 (23)	Indirect, oscillometric	>160	164–325	Barthez et al, 1997[71]
	3 (5)	Indirect, Doppler	>160	135–214	Kook et al, in press[70]

onset and usually takes months to years to produce full-blown signs (eg, polyuria, polydipsia, polyphagia, pendulous abdomen, panting, alopecia, or muscle and skin atrophy).

In people, hypertension is a common complication with a reported prevalence of between 55% and 80%.[37–39] The hypertension is characterized by disruption of the circadian rhythm of blood pressure, with loss of the physiologic nocturnal fall.[40] Mortality rate is increased because the risk of cardiovascular disease is four to five times higher than the population average.[38,41] The mechanisms by which glucocorticoids are involved in the etiology of hypertension are (1) their intrinsic mineralocorticoid activity; (2) activation of the renin-angiotensin-aldosterone system; (3) enhancement of cardiovascular inotropic and pressor activity of vasoactive substances, including catecholamines or vasopressin and angiotensin II; and (4) suppression of the vasodilatory system, including the nitric oxide (NO) synthase, prostacyclin, and kinin–kallikrein systems.[42–45] Recently, a large body of evidence has implicated the NO system in glucocorticoid-induced hypertension. Glucocorticoids interact with, and impair, the NO pathway by (1) down-regulation of NO synthase synthesis, (2) impairment of the L-arginine transport system, and (3) suppression of tetrahydrobiopterin synthesis, which is a cofactor for NO synthase.[46–48]

The occurrence of hypertension in dogs with hyperadrenocorticism has been documented in several studies (see **Table 3**).[4,49–53] The prevalence is similar to that reported in humans and ranges from 59% to 86%.[50,51] Systemic hypertension was most prevalent and blood pressure was highest in dogs with an untreated adrenocortical tumor.[51] At the authors' clinic, the current prevalence of hypertension (systolic blood pressure $\geq$ 150 mm Hg) in dogs with hyperadrenocorticism is 78%; 58% have blood pressure values of between 150 and 179 mm Hg, which is considered a mild to moderate risk, and 42% have blood pressure values greater than or equal to 180 mm Hg, which is considered a severe risk of target-organ damage. Sequelae of hypertension in dogs with hyperadrenocorticism have been limited to the eyes and kidneys. Proteinuria, as a marker for renal damage, has been reported to range from 44% to 75%.[51,54] Development of blindness from intraocular hemorrhage and retinal detachment has been reported by Littman and colleagues.[49]

The mechanisms involved in the development of hypertension in dogs with hyperadrenocorticism have not been elucidated. The role of aldosterone was recently investigated but the results are conflicting. Nine of 13 dogs with pituitary-dependent hyperadrenocorticism (PDH) had a systolic blood pressure greater than 200 mm Hg. Plasma aldosterone concentrations were lower in affected dogs before and after corticotropin stimulation compared with normal dogs, which suggests that aldosterone is not involved.[52] Similar findings were reported in a study by Javadi and colleagues,[55] in which mean basal plasma aldosterone concentrations were significantly lower in 31 dogs with PDH than in 12 healthy dogs. These results are in contrast to findings of a study in which aldosterone concentrations in 17 dogs with PDH were significantly higher than aldosterone concentrations in 12 healthy dogs.[56]

Martinez and colleagues[57] demonstrated increased vascular reactivity to increasing doses of norepinephrine in dogs with experimentally induced hypercortisolism. Norepinephrine resulted in severe hypertension (systolic blood pressure >240 mm Hg) in seven of eight dogs with iatrogenic hypercortisolism but in only three of eight control dogs. The authors recently showed that glucocorticoids activate the endothelin system. Dogs with experimentally induced hypercortisolism had significantly higher plasma concentrations of endothelin-1 compared with control dogs. In contrast to current data in human medicine, there was no evidence to support reduced NO availability as a cause of increased blood pressure. Because blood pressure was only mildly increased, however, it is possible that the role of NOS synthesis was masked.[58,59]

A significant proportion of dogs remain hypertensive despite adequate control of excessive glucocorticoids. In one study, 40% of dogs with well-controlled hyperadrenocorticism were hypertensive, which is similar to the percentage of well-managed people.[51,60] In Goy-Thollot and colleagues[52] study, the prevalence of persistent hypertension was not reported, but blood pressure values in dogs treated with o,p'-DDD for 3 months were still significantly higher than those of control dogs.

In human medicine, persistent hypertension is treated with substances belonging to various classes of drugs, including angiotensin II receptor blockers, angiotensin-converting enzyme inhibitors, and aldosterone antagonists. The use of these drugs in dogs with persistent hypertension despite adequate control of hyperadrenocorticism needs to be evaluated.

PHEOCHROMOCYTOMA

Pheochromocytoma is a catecholamine-secreting neuroendocrine tumor, which is uncommon in dogs and rare in cats. In the normal adrenal medulla of dogs, cats, and humans, 60% to 80% of the catecholamine content is epinephrine, which is, therefore, the major catecholamine.[61] In human pheochromocytomas, norepinephrine is the predominant catecholamine secreted and in some tumors it may be the only catecholamine produced. On rare occasions, tumors may secrete only epinephrine.[62] The secretory patterns of canine and feline pheochromocytomas have not yet been investigated.

Norepinephrine and epinephrine interact with α- and β-adrenergic receptors. Compared with norepinephrine, however, epinephrine has a higher affinity for adrenergic receptors in general and β_2-adrenergic receptors in particular and is more potent. **Table 4** lists catecholamine receptor types, subtypes, and adrenergic responses. Hypertension is mainly the result of excessive stimulation of α_1 and β_1 receptors.

The clinical presentation of animals with pheochromocytoma is highly variable and ranges from complete absence of signs to dramatic and life-threatening signs; the

Table 4		
Catecholamine receptor types and subtypes and adrenergic responses		
Organ/Tissue	**Receptor Type**	**Effect**
Cardiovascular system	β_1	Increase in heart rate, increase in contractility
	α_1	Vasoconstriction
	β_2	Vasodilation in skeletal muscle arterioles, coronary arteries and all veins
Bronchial muscles	β_2	Relaxation
Gastrointestinal tract	β_2	Decrease in motility
Pancreatic islets	α_2	Decrease in insulin and glucagon secretion
	β_2	Increase in insulin and glucagon secretion
Liver	β_2	Increase in glycogenolysis and gluconeogenesis
Adipose tissue	β_2	Increase in lipolysis
Urinary bladder	α_2	Increase in sphincter tone
	β_2	Relaxation of detrusor muscle
Eye	α_1	Mydriasis

latter are usually the result of a hypertensive crisis. Clinical signs depend on the type of catecholamine produced by the tumor and the amount and frequency of catecholamine release into the circulation. Clinical signs are usually episodic; they may occur several times per day or may only recur after weeks or months (**Table 5**).

Ninety percent to 95% of human patients with pheochromocytoma have hypertension. Blood pressure patterns vary: approximately 50% of patients have sustained hypertension with marked fluctuations and severe episodic blood pressure peaks; approximately 25% are normotensive between hypertensive episodes; and the remaining patients have stable and sustained hypertension.[61,63–65] Hypertension varies from mild to severe (eg, systolic blood pressure >250 mm Hg),[66] and the systolic rise during a hypertensive paroxysm may be up to 200 mm Hg.[67] Episodic hypotension or even syncope may occur in patients with tumors that secrete mainly epinephrine.[61]

Although lesions attributable to hypertension were described decades ago in dogs with pheochromocytoma,[68] blood pressure was not measured in most of the cases. Current information on blood pressure values is limited to fewer than 50 dogs, approximately half of which had hypertension.[69–74] Similar to the situation in human medicine, the increase in blood pressure in dogs may range from mild to severe; the maximum systolic pressure reported was 325 mm Hg (see **Table 3**).[69]

Fluctuations in blood pressure that occur in dogs with pheochromocytoma cannot be determined from the studies published, although in some dogs blood pressure was measured on several occasions. In the authors' most recent study, blood pressure patterns in dogs and humans were assumed to be similar. Two of five dogs with pheochromocytoma had multiple systolic blood pressure measurements, which were always less than 160 mm Hg. Variable paroxysmal hypertensive peaks with systolic values of 270 mm Hg occurred in one dog, and marked fluctuations of systolic pressure from 55 to 175 mm Hg and a single episode of increased systolic pressure of 180 mm Hg were seen in the two others.[70]

Diagnosis of pheochromocytoma can be challenging and may require diagnostic imaging and measurement of urinary metanephrines.[75] Adrenalectomy is the treatment of choice; however, there is a high risk of hypertensive and hypotensive crises, cardiac arrhythmias, and hemorrhage.[76–78] Surgery should be performed only by a team of experienced surgeons and an anesthetist. In humans, α-adrenergic blockade (usually phenoxybenzamine) is used for at least 1 week before

Table 5	
Clinical signs in dogs with pheochromocytoma	
Categories of Clinical Symptoms	**Symptoms**
Unspecific	Anorexia, weight loss, lethargy
Related to cardiorespiratory system and/or hypertension	Tachypnea; panting; tachycardia; arrhythmias; collapse; pale mucus membranes; nasal-, gingival-, ocular hemorrhage; acute blindness
Related to neuromuscular system	Weakness, anxiety, pacing, muscle tremor, seizures
Miscellaneous	Polyuria/polydipsia, vomiting, diarrhea, painful abdomen
Related to large, malignant tumor	Abdominal distension, ascites, hind-limb edema, intra-abdominal or retroperitoneal hemorrhage

adrenalectomy. The aim is to reverse vasoconstriction and hypovolemia and control fluctuations of blood pressure and heart rate during anesthesia. The recommended starting dosage of phenoxybenzamine in dogs is 0.25 mg/kg twice a day, which is gradually increased every few days until signs of hypotension or adverse drug reaction occur or a maximum dosage of 2.5 mg/kg twice a day is attained.[79] A recent study showed that although there was no difference in intra- and postoperative hypo- and hypertensive episodes and arrhythmias, dogs treated with phenoxybenzamine had significantly decreased mortality compared with untreated dogs.[78] In cases in which adrenalectomy is not an option, phenoxybenzamine should be used on a long-term basis to control blood pressure. Additional β-adrenergic therapy may be necessary in patients with severe tachycardia, but it should not be given without prior α-blockade to avoid severe hypertension.

HYPERTHYROIDISM

Hyperthyroidism is the most common feline endocrine disease with an estimated prevalence of 2%[80] but is rare in dogs. More than 98% of cats with hyperthyroidism have adenomatous hyperplasia or adenoma; thyroid carcinoma is uncommon.[81] Characteristic clinical signs include polyphagia with simultaneous weight loss; polyuria; polydipsia; behavioral changes, such as restlessness or aggressiveness; and vomiting and diarrhea. Some cats have atypical signs, such as anorexia and lethargy.

In hyperthyroid humans, excessive levels of circulating thyroxine cause a 40% to 60% decrease in systemic vascular resistance. This decline is accompanied by a decrease in diastolic blood pressure, which in turn causes a reflex increase in heart rate, stroke volume, and cardiac output. The effect of these changes on renal physiology is considerable: a fall in systemic vascular resistance induces a decline in renal perfusion pressure, and this stimulates the release of renin, leading to increased production of angiotensin. This may partly explain the high levels of angiotensin-converting enzyme in hyperthyroidism. The sum of these changes is augmentation of renal sodium reabsorption and expansion of total body sodium content and blood volume.[82,83] An excess of thyroid hormones also leads to increased sensitivity to circulating catecholamines resulting in direct induction of inotropy and chronotropy. Systolic arterial pressure is almost always increased in human patients with hyperthyroidism.[84] The disease usually has only minor effects on mean arterial pressure, however, because the increase in systolic blood pressure is offset by the decrease in diastolic pressure.[85] These changes lead to increased pulse pressure typical of hyperthyroidism.[84] In addition to systemic hypertension, hyperthyroidism may cause pulmonary hypertension. Several reports describe hyperthyroidism and concomitant pulmonary hypertension with resolution of the latter after treatment of the hyperthyroid state.[86] The mechanisms leading to hypertension in feline hyperthyroidism have not been investigated in detail but are presumably similar to those described in human medicine.

The prevalence of systemic hypertension in the hyperthyroid feline population is estimated to be between 5% and 22%.[87–90] Alternatively, a prevalence of 9% has been found for hyperthyroidism in hypertensive cats.[91] The number may have been underestimated in the latter study, however, because serum thyroxine concentrations were only determined in half of the cats. Severe hypertension has been considered uncommon in feline hyperthyroidism[10,92,93] and the most recent studies support this affirmation with reported median values of 140 to 186 mm Hg.[87,88,94–96] If severe hypertension is documented, concomitant diseases, such as renal failure, should be suspected.[10,97,98] Unfortunately, chronic kidney disease may be masked at initial presentation because the increased glomerular filtration rate induced by hyperthyroidism maintains serum urea and creatinine concentrations in the reference range. Azotemia, therefore, only becomes obvious after hyperthyroidism is treated. This is estimated to occur in approximately 17% to 39% of cats.[96,99–102]

The effect of restoration of euthyroidism on blood pressure has been evaluated in several studies of cats with hyperthyroidism. In most studies no significant changes in blood pressure were detected during treatment for hyperthyroidism, independent of the therapeutic option chosen.[87,88,94,96,103] Syme and Elliot[93] demonstrated a significant decrease in blood pressure, however, after initiation of treatment with carbimazole or thyroidectomy. In the latter study, 22.5% of the cats with well-controlled hyperthyroidism had been normotensive at the time of diagnosis but developed hypertension during treatment. This observation is supported by a recent study in which 22.8% of cats with hyperthyroidism were normotensive initially but developed hypertension after re-establishment of euthyroidism with medical or surgical treatment.[90] Based on these reports, the majority of initially hypertensive hyperthyroid cats, and all cats that develop hypertension after restoration of euthyroidism, need additional medication to control blood pressure. The β-blocker atenolol was ineffective as a single antihypertensive drug in 70% of hyperthyroid cats,[95] and addition of an angiotensin-converting enzyme inhibitor or amlodipine besylate is generally required. Because of the high incidence of hypertension after restoration of euthyroidism, monitoring of blood pressure is recommended during therapy, independent of the treatment option.

DIABETES MELLITUS

Diabetes mellitus is one of the most common endocrine diseases in humans and in dogs and cats. In diabetic people, hypertension is a frequently encountered comorbid condition, affecting 10% to 30% of patients with type 1 and 30% to 50% of patients with type 2 diabetes mellitus.[104] The relationship between diabetes and hypertension is complex. Not only are diabetics prone to hypertension but also hypertensive patients are at risk of developing diabetes.[105] The risk for stroke or cardiovascular disease is two times higher and the risk for end-stage renal disease is five to six times higher in patients with hypertension and diabetes than in nondiabetic patients with hypertension.

In human type 1 diabetes, hypertension is usually a manifestation of diabetic nephropathy, each of which exacerbates the other. In human patients with type 2 diabetes, hypertension is assumed to be associated with other features of metabolic syndrome, such as insulin resistance, hyperlipidemia, and central obesity.[104,106] Possible causes of hypertension are loss of the normal vasodilator effect of insulin (eg, loss of insulin-induced NO generation), increase in sodium and water retention, increase in intracellular calcium concentration enhancing contractility of vascular smooth muscle, proliferation of vascular smooth muscle, and stimulation of sympathetic outflow.[107,108]

Information on blood pressure in diabetic dogs and cats is scarce. Bodey and Michell[4] found blood pressure higher in a group of dogs with diabetes mellitus compared with a group of healthy dogs. That study did not mention, however, whether or not the dogs were truly hypertensive. In another study, blood pressure was higher in eight dogs with recently diagnosed diabetes than in 40 healthy control dogs. Only one of the eight, however, was slightly hypertensive.[109] It is possible that hypertension is of greater importance in dogs with long-standing diabetes. In 50 dogs treated for diabetes for a median of 6 months, hypertension was detected in 23 (46%), a number that compares to the prevalence in human diabetics. Blood pressure was higher in dogs with longer duration of diabetes, and hypertension was associated with increased albumin excretion in the urine.[110] The clinical relevance of those findings, including the risk of diabetic dogs developing kidney damage, is currently unknown and deserves further investigation.

There is currently no convincing evidence that diabetic cats have hypertension. Of eight cats with recently diagnosed diabetes, two had increased systolic blood pressure of 170 and 180 mm Hg. Values of 170 and 180 mm Hg, however, were also found in 2 of 20 healthy control cats.[111] Similar findings were described in 14 cats with a median diabetes duration of 18 months. None of the cats had systolic blood pressures greater than 180 mm Hg, and blood pressures of healthy controls and diabetic cats did not differ. None of the cats had proteinuria or retinopathy.[112] These findings are in agreement with two other studies, in which the duration of diabetes was not specified; however, none of the 13 cats examined had hypertension.[113,114] Nevertheless, there may be single exceptional cases. In one study, two diabetic cats with hypertensive retinopathy were described; one had evidence of renal dysfunction, which may have been the cause of hypertension, but the other cat had no other known concurrent disease.[9] Further studies using larger cohorts of diabetic cats are needed to evaluate questions, such as the definitive prevalence of hypertension and the risk of kidney damage when blood pressure is in the upper end of normal.

OTHER ENDOCRINE DISORDERS

In human medicine, other endocrine disorders have been associated with hypertension, including hypothyroidism, primary hyperparathyroidism, and acromegaly. To date, there are no reports of hypertension associated with these diseases in dogs and cats.

REFERENCES

1. Chobanian AV, Bakris GL, Black HR, et al. The seventh report of the joint national committee on prevention, detection, evaluation, and treatment of high blood pressure. Hypertension 2003;42:1206–52.
2. Black HR. The paradigm has shifted to systolic blood pressure. J Hum Hypertens 2004;18:3–7.
3. Brown S, Atkins C, Bagley R, et al. Guidelines for the identification, evaluation, and management of systemic hypertension in dogs and cats. J Vet Intern Med 2007;21:542–58.
4. Bodey AR, Michell AR. Epidemiological study of blood pressure in domestic dogs. J Small Anim Pract 1996;37(3):116–25.
5. Brown SA. Pathophysiology of systemic hypertension. In: Ettinger SJ, Feldman EC, editors, Textbook of veterinary internal medicine. Diseases of the dog and cat, vol. I. 6th edition. St. Louis (MO): Elsevier Saunders; 2005. p. 472–6.
6. Anderson GH, Blakeman N, Streeten DH. The effect of age on prevalence of secondary forms of hypertension in 4429 consecutively referred patients. J Hypertens 1994;12(5):609–15.
7. Stowasser M, Gordon RD, Gunasekera TG, et al. High rate of detection of primary hyperaldosteronism, including surgically treatable forms, after 'nonselective' screening of hypertensive patients. J Hypertens 2003;21(11):2149–57.

8. Omura M, Saito J, Yamaguchi K, et al. Prospective study on the prevalence of secondary hypertension among hypertensive patients visiting a general outpatient clinic in Japan. Hypertens Res 2004;27(3):193–202.
9. Maggio F, DeFrancesco TC, Atkins CE, et al. Ocular lesions associated with systemic hypertension in cats: 69 cases (1985–1998). J Am Vet Med Assoc 2000;217(5):695–702.
10. Elliott J, Barber PJ, Syme HM, et al. Feline hypertension: clinical findings and response to antihypertensive treatment in 30 cases. J Small Anim Pract 2001; 42:122–9.
11. Mishina M, Watanabe T, Matsuoka S, et al. Diurnal variations of blood pressure in dogs. J Vet Med Sci 1999;61:643–7.
12. Piccione G, Grasso F, Giudice E. Circadian rhythm in the cardiovascular system of domestic animals. Res Vet Sci 2005;79:155–60.
13. Gosse P, Promax H, Durandet P, et al. 'White coat' hypertension. No harm for the heart. Hypertension 1993;22:766–70.
14. Schellenberg S, Glaus TM, Reusch CE. Effect of long-term adaptation on indirect measurements of systolic blood pressure in conscious untrained beagles. Vet Rec 2007;161:418–21.
15. Kaplan NM. Hypertensive and atherosclerotic cardiovascular disease. In: Braunwald E, Libby P, editors. Heart disease. 6th edition. Philadelphia: WB Saunders Company; 2001. p. 941–71.
16. Eger CE, Robinson WF, Huxtable CR. Primary hyperhyperaldosteronism (Conn's syndrome) in a cat: a case report and review of comparative aspects. J Soc Adm Pharm 1983;24:293–307.
17. Breitschwerdt EB, Meuten DJ, Greenfield CL, et al. Idiopathic hyperaldosteronism in a dog. J Am Vet Med Assoc 1985;187:841–5.
18. Rijnberk A, Kooistra HS, van Vonderen IK, et al. Aldosteronoma in a dog with polyuria as the leading symptom. Domest Anim Endocrinol 2001;20:227–40.
19. Johnson KD, Henry CJ, McCaw DL, et al. Primary hyperaldosteronism in a dog with concurrent lymphoma. J Vet Med 2006;53:467–70.
20. Feldman EC, Nelson RW. Primary mineralocorticoid excess-primary hyperhyperaldosteronism. In: Feldman EC, Nelson RW, editors. Canine and feline endocrinology and reproduction. 3rd edition. Philadelphia: WB Saunders; 2004. p. 351–7.
21. Young WF. Primary hyperaldosteronism: renaissance of a syndrome. Clin Endocrinol 2007;66:607–18.
22. Mulatero P, Stowasser M, Loh KC, et al. Increased diagnosis of primary hyperaldosteronism, including surgically correctable forms, in centers from five continents. J Clin Endocrinol Metab 2004;89:1045–50.
23. Gordon RD, Laragh JH, Funder JW. Low renin hypertensive states: perspectives, unsolved problems, future research. Trends Endocrinol Metab 2005;16:108 13.
24. Gaddam KK, Pimenta E, Husain S, et al. Aldosterone and cardiovascular disease. Curr Probl Cardiol 2009;34:51–84.
25. Rossi GP, Bernini G, Desideri G, et al. Renal damage in primary hyperaldosteronism: results of the PAPY study. Hypertension 2006;48:232–8.
26. Milliez P, Girerd X, Plouin PF, et al. Evidence for an increased rate of cardiovascular events in patients with primary hyperaldosteronism. J Am Coll Cardiol 2005;45:1243–8.
27. Fallo F, Veglio F, Bertello C, et al. Prevalence and characteristics of the metabolic syndrome in primary hyperaldosteronism. J Clin Endocrinol Metab 2006;91: 454–9.

28. MacKay AD, Holt PE, Sparkes AH. Successful surgical treatment of a cat with primary hyperaldosteronism. J Feline Med Surg 1999;1:117–22.
29. Flood SM, Randolph JF, Gelzer AR, et al. Primary hyperaldosteronism in two cats. J Am Anim Hosp Assoc 1999;35:411–6.
30. Moore LE, Biller DS, Smith TA. Use of abdominal ultrasonography in the diagnosis of primary hyperaldosteronism in a cat. J Am Vet Med Assoc 2000;217: 213–5.
31. Rijnberk A, Voorhout G, Kooistra HS, et al. Hyperaldosteronism in a cat with metastasised adrenocortical tumour. Vet Q 2001;23:38–43.
32. DeClue AE, Breshears LA, Pardo ID, et al. Hyperaldosteronism and hyperprogesteronism in a cat with an adrenal cortical carcinoma. J Vet Intern Med 2005;19:355–8.
33. Rose SA, Kyles AE, Labelle P, et al. Adrenalectomy and caval thrombectomy in a cat with primary hyperaldosteronism. J Am Anim Hosp Assoc 2007;43: 209–14.
34. Renschler JS, Dean GA. What is your diagnosis? Abdominal mass aspirate in a cat with an increased Na:K ratio. Vet Clin Pathol 2009;38:69–72.
35. Ash RA, Harvey AM, Tasker S. Primary hyperaldosteronism in the cat: a series of 13 cases. J Feline Med Surg 2005;7:173–82.
36. Javady S, Djajadiningrat-Laanen SC, Kooistra HS, et al. Primary hyperaldosteronism, a mediator of progressive renal disease in cats. Domest Anim Endocrinol 2005;28:85–104.
37. Melby JC. Clinical review 1: endocrine hypertension. J Clin Endocrinol Metab 1989;69:697–703.
38. Etxabe J, Vazquez JA. Morbidity and mortality in Cushing's disease: an epidemiological approach. Clin Endocrinol (Oxf) 1994;40:479–84.
39. Boscaro M, Barzon L, Fallo F, et al. Cushing's syndrome. Lancet 2001;357: 783–91.
40. Imai Y, Abe K, Sasaki S, et al. Altered circadian blood pressure rhythm in patients with Cushing's syndrome. Hypertension 1988;12:11–9.
41. Ross EJ, Linch DC. Cushing's syndrome—killing disease: discriminatory value of signs and symptoms aiding early diagnosis. Lancet 1982;2:646–9.
42. Suzuki H, Handa M, Kondo K, et al. Role of renin-angiotensin system in glucocorticoid hypertension in rats. Am J Phys 1982;243:E48–51.
43. Saruta T, Suzuki H, Handa M, et al. Multiple factors contribute to the pathogenesis of hypertension in Cushing's syndrome. J Clin Endocrinol Metab 1986;62: 275–9.
44. Kelly JJ, Tam SH, Williamson PM, et al. The nitric oxide system and cortisol-induced hypertension in humans. Clin Exp Pharmacol Physiol 1998;25:945–6.
45. Heaney AP, Hunter SJ, Sheridan B, et al. Increased pressor response to noradrenaline in pituitary dependent Cushing's syndrome. Clin Endocrinol (Oxf) 1999;51:293–9.
46. Radomski MW, Palmer RM, Moncada S. Glucocorticoids inhibit the expression of an inducible, but not the constitutive, nitric oxide synthase in vascular endothelial cells. Proc Natl Acad Sci U S A 1990;87:1043–7.
47. Simmons WW, Ungureanu-Longrois D, Smith GK, et al. Glucocorticoids regulate inducible nitric oxide synthase by inhibiting tetrahydrobiopterin synthesis and L-arginine transport. J Biol Chem 1996;271:23928–37.
48. Mitchell BM, Dorrance AM, Webb RC. GTP cyclohydrolase 1 downregulation contributes to glucocorticoid hypertension in rats. Hypertension 2003;41: 669–74.

49. Littman MP, Robertson JL, Bovee KC. Spontaneous systemic hypertension in dogs: five cases (1981–1983). J Am Vet Med Assoc 1988;193:486–94.
50. Cowgill LD. Clinical significance, diagnosis and management of hypertension in dogs and cats. Partners in practice (Hill's Pet Products) 1991;4:2–3.
51. Ortega TM, Feldman EC, Nelson RW, et al. Systemic arterial blood pressure and urine protein/creatinine ratio in dogs with hyperadrenocorticism. J Am Vet Med Assoc 1996;209:1724–9.
52. Goy-Thollot I, Pechereau D, Keroack S, et al. Investigation of the role of aldosterone in hypertension associated with spontaneous pituitary-dependent hyperadrenocorticism in dogs. J Small Anim Pract 2002;43:489–92.
53. Novellas R, de Gopegui RR, Espada Y. Determination of renal vascular resistance in dogs with diabetes mellitus and hyperadrenocorticism. Vet Rec 2008; 163:592–6.
54. Hurley KJ, Vaden SL. Evaluation of urine protein content in dogs with pituitary-dependent hyperadrenocorticism. J Am Vet Med Assoc 1998;212:369–73.
55. Javadi S, Kooistra HS, Mol JA, et al. Plasma aldosterone concentrations and plasma renin activity in healthy dogs and dogs with hyperadrenocorticism. Vet Rec 2003;153:521–5.
56. Wenger M, Sieber-Ruckstuhl NS, Müller C, et al. Effect of trilostane on serum concentrations of aldosterone, cortisol, and potassium in dogs with pituitary-dependent hyperadrenocorticism. Am J Vet Res 2004;65:1245–50.
57. Martinez NI, Panciera DL, Abbott JA, et al. Evaluation of pressor sensitivity to norepinephrine infusion in dogs with iatrogenic hyperadrenocorticism. Pressor sensitivity in dogs with hyperadrenocorticism. Res Vet Sci 2005;78:25–31.
58. Schellenberg S, Reusch CE, Glaus TM. Role of cardiovascular peptides in cortisol-induced hypertension in dogs [abstract 77]. In: Congress Proceedings ECVIM Forum. Amsterdam; 2006. p. 178.
59. Schellenberg S, Kleinbongard P, Kelm M, et al. The nitric oxide system in hydrocortisone-induced hypertension in dogs [abstract 240]. In: Proceedings ACVIM Forum. Seattle; 2007. p. 834.
60. Simon D, Goretzki PE, Lollert A, et al. Persistent hypertension after successful adrenal operation. Surgery 1993;114:1189–95.
61. Fitzgerald PA, Goldfien A. Adrenal medulla. In: Greenspan FS, Gardner DG, editors. Basic & clinical endocrinology. 7th edition. New York: Lange Medical Books/McGraw-Hill; 2004. p. 439–77.
62. Hsueh WA, Nicholas SB, Hamaty M, et al. Endocrinology of hypertension. In: Felig P, Frohmann LA, editors. Endocrinology and metabolism. 4th edition. New York: McGraw-Hill Inc; 2001. p. 553–608.
63. Young WF. Endocrine hypertension. In: Kronenberg HM, Melmed S, Polonsky KS, et al, editors. Williams textbook of endocrinology. Philadelphia: Saunders Elsevier; 2008. p. 505–37.
64. Fountoulakis S, Tsatsoulis A. Molecular genetic aspects and pathophysiology of endocrine hypertension. Hormones 2006;5(2):90–106.
65. Kopetschke R, Slisko M, Kilisli A, et al. Frequent incidental discovery of pheochromocytoma - data from a German cohort of 201 pheochromocytoma. Eur J Endocrinol 2009;161(2):355–61.
66. Lentschener C, Gaujoux S, Thillois JM, et al. Increased arterial pressure is not predictive of haemodynamic instability in patients undergoing adrenalectomy for pheochromocytoma. Acta Anaesthesiol Scand 2009;53:522–7.
67. Manelli M, Ianni L, Cilotti A. Pheochromocytoma in Italy: a multicentric retrospective study. Eur J Endocrinol 1999;141:619–24.

68. Howard EB, Nielsen SW. Pheochromocytomas associated with hypertensive lesions in dogs. J Am Vet Med Assoc 1965;147(3):245–52.
69. Gilson SD, Withrow SJ, Wheeler SL, et al. Pheochromocytoma in 50 dogs. J Vet Intern Med 1994;8:228–32.
70. Kook PH, Grest P, Quante S, et al. Urinary catecholamine and metanephrine to creatinine ratios in 7 dogs with pheochromocytoma. Vet Rec, in press.
71. Barthez PY, Marks SL, Woo J, et al. Pheochromocytoma in dogs: 61 cases (1984–1995). J Vet Intern Med 1997;11(5):272–8.
72. Williams JE, Hackner SG. Pheochromocytoma presenting as acute retroperitoneal hemorrhage in a dog. J Vet Emerg Crit Care 2001;11(3):221–7.
73. Whittemore JC, Preston CA, Kyles AE, et al. Nontraumatic rupture of an adrenal gland tumor causing intra-abdominal or retroperitoneal hemorrhage in four dogs. J Am Vet Med Assoc 2001;219(3):329–33.
74. Brown AJ, Alwood AJ, Cole SG, et al. Malignant pheochromocytoma presenting as a bradyarrhythmia in a dog. J Vet Emerg Crit Care 2007;17(2):164–9.
75. Kook PH, Boretti FS, Hersberger M, et al. Urinary catecholamine and metanephrine to creatinine ratios in healthy dogs at home and in a hospital environment and in 2 dogs with pheochromocytoma. J Vet Intern Med 2007;21:388–93.
76. Gilson SD, Withrow SJ, Orton EC. Surgical treatment of pheochromocytoma: technique, complications, and results in six dogs. Vet Surg 1994;23:195–200.
77. Wright KN, Feldman JM, Meuten DJ, et al. Diagnostic and therapeutic considerations in a hypercalcemic dog with multiple endocrine neoplasia. J Am Anim Hosp Assoc 1995;31:156–62.
78. Herrera MA, Mehl ML, Kass PH, et al. Predictive factors and the effect of phenoxybenzamine on outcome in dogs undergoing adrenalectomy for pheochromocytoma. J Vet Intern Med 2008;22:1333–9.
79. Feldman EC, Nelson RW. Pheochromocytoma and multiple endocrine neoplasia. In: Feldman EC, Nelson RW, editors. Canine and feline endocrinology and reproduction. 3rd edition. St. Louis (MO): Saunders; 2004. p. 440–63.
80. Edinboro CH, Scott-Moncrieff JC, Janovitz E, et al. Epidemiologic study of relationships between consumption of commercial canned food and risk of hyperthyroidism in cats. J Am Vet Med Assoc 2004;224:879–86.
81. Peterson ME, Ward CR. Etiopathologic findings of hyperthyroidism in cats. Vet Clin North Am Small Anim Pract 2007;37:633–45.
82. Klein I, Ojamaa K. Thyrotoxicosis and the heart. Endocrinol Metab Clin North Am 1998;27:51–62.
83. Lozano HF, Sharma CN. Reversible pulmonary hypertension, tricuspid regurgitation and right-sided heart failure associated with hyperthyroidism. Case report and review of the literature. Cardiol Rev 2004;12:299–305.
84. Fazio S, Palmieri EA, Lombardi G, et al. Effects of thyroid hormone on the cardiovascular system. Recent Prog Horm Res 2004;59:31–50.
85. Polikar R, Burger AG, Scherrer U, et al. The thyroid and the heart. Circulation 1993;87:1435–41.
86. Hegazi MO, El Sayed A, El Ghoussein H. Pulmonary hypertension responding to hyperthyroidism treatment. Respirology 2008;13:923–5.
87. Trepanier LA, Hoffman SB, Kroll M, et al. Efficacy and safety of once versus twice daily administration of methimazole in cats with hyperthyroidism. J Am Vet Med Assoc 2003;222:954–8.
88. Sartor LL, Trepanier LA, Kroll MM, et al. Efficacy and safety of transdermal methimazole in the treatment of cats with hyperthyroidism. J Vet Intern Med 2004; 18:651–5.

89. Trepanier LA. Pharmacologic management of feline hyperthyroidism. Vet Clin North Am Small Anim Pract 2007;37:775–88.

90. Morrow LD, Adams VJ, Elliott J, et al. Hypertension in hyperthyroid cats: prevalence, incidence, and predictors of its development. J Vet Intern Med 2009;23:699.

91. Chetboul V, Lefebvre HP, Pinhas C, et al. Spontaneous feline hypertension: clinical and echocardiographic abnormalities, and survival rate. J Vet Intern Med 2003;17:89–95.

92. van der Woerdt A, Peterson ME. Prevalence of ocular abnormalities in cats with hyperthyroidism. J Vet Intern Med 2000;14:202–3.

93. Syme HM, Elliott J. The prevalence of hypertension in hyperthyroid cats at diagnosis and following treatment. J Vet Intern Med 2003;17:754.

94. Stepien RL, Rapoport GS, Henik RA, et al. Effect of measurement method on blood pressure findings in cats before and after therapy for hyperthyroidism. J Vet Intern Med 2003;17:754.

95. Henik RA, Stepien RL, Wenholz LJ, et al. Efficacy of atenolol as a single antihypertensive agent in hyperthyroid cats. J Feline Med Surg 2008;10:577–82.

96. van Hoek I, Lefebvre HP, Peremans K, et al. Short- and long-term follow-up of glomerular and tubular renal markers of kidney function in hyperthyroid cats after treatment with radioiodine. Domest Anim Endocrinol 2009;36:45–56.

97. Littman MP. Spontaneous systemic hypertension in 24 cats. J Vet Intern Med 1994;8:79–86.

98. Stiles J, Polzind DJ, Bistner SI. The prevalence of retinopathy in cats with systemic hypertension and chronic renal failure or hyperthyroidism. J Am Anim Hosp Assoc 1994;30:564–72.

99. Graves TK, Olivier NB, Nachreiner RF, et al. Changes in renal function associated with treatment of hyperthyroidism in cats. Am J Vet Res 1994;55:1745–9.

100. Becker TJ, Graves TK, Kruger JM, et al. Effects of methimazole on renal function in cats with hyperthyroidism. J Am Anim Hosp Assoc 2000;36:215–23.

101. Milner RJ, Channell CD, Levy JK, et al. Survival times for cats with hyperthyroidism treated with iodine 131, methimazole, or both: 167 cases (1996–2003). J Am Vet Med Assoc 2006;228:559–63.

102. Langston CE, Reine NJ. Hyperthyroidism and the kidney. Clin Tech Small Anim Pract 2006;21:17–21.

103. Boag AK, Neiger R, Slater L, et al. Changes in the glomerular filtration rate of 27 cats with hyperthyroidism after treatment with radioactive iodine. Vet Rec 2007; 161:711–5.

104. Nilsson PM. Hypertension in diabetes mellitus. In: Pickup JC, Williams G, editors. Textbook of diabetes. 3rd edition. St. Louis (MO), Massachusetts: Blackwell Science; 2003. p. 51.1-51.22.

105. McFarlane SI, Castro J, Kirpichnikov D, et al. Hypertension in diabetes mellitus. In: Kahn CR, King GL, Moses AC, et al, editors. Joslin's diabetes mellitus. 14th edition. Philadelphia: Lippincott Williams & Wilkins; 2005. p. 969–74.

106. Huang PL. A comprehensive definition for metabolic syndrome. Dis Model Mech 2009;2:231–7.

107. DeFronzo RA, Ferrannini E. Insulin resistance. A multifaceted syndrome responsible for NIDDM, obesity, hypertension, dyslipidemia, and atherosclerotic cardiovascular disease. Diabetes Care 1991;14(3):173–94.

108. Weidmann P, deCourten M, Böhlen L. Insulin resistance, hyperinsulinemia and hypertension. J Hypertens Suppl 1993;11(5):27–38.

109. Kolb S. Indirekte Blutdruckmessung bei gesunden Hunden, Hunden mit Cushing-Syndrom, Diabetes Mellitus und chronischer Nephropathie. Inaugural-

Dissertation zur Erlangung der tiermedizinischen Doktorwürde der Tierärztlichen Fakultät der Ludwig-Maximilians-Universität München [dissertation]. 2000.

110. Struble AL, Feldman EC, Nelson RW, et al. Systemic hypertension and proteinuria in dogs with diabetes mellitus. J Am Vet Med Assoc 1998;213(6):822–5.

111. Sander C. Indirekte Blutdruckmessung mit der oszillometrischen und der Doppler-sonographischen Methode bei gesunden Katzen und bei Katzen mit Diabetes Mellitus, chronischer Nephropathie und hypertropher Kardiomyopathie. Inaugural-Dissertation zur Erlangung der tiermedizinischen Doktorwürde der Tierärztlichen Fakultät der Ludwig-Maximilians-Universität München [dissertation]. 1997.

112. Sennello KA, Schulman RL, Prosek R, et al. Systolic blood pressure in cats with diabetes mellitus. J Am Vet Med Assoc 2003;223(2):198–201.

113. Bodey AR, Sansom J. Epidemiological study of blood pressure in domestic cats. J Small Anim Pract 1998;39:567–73.

114. Norris CR, Nelson RW, Christopher MM. Serum total and ionized magnesium concentrations and urinary fractional excretion of magnesium in cats with diabetes mellitus and diabetic ketoacidosis. J Am Vet Med Assoc 1999;215(10): 1455–9.

Feline Primary Hyperaldosteronism

Rhonda L. Schulman, DVM

KEYWORDS

- Primary hyperaldosteronism • Primary aldosteronism
- Conn's disease • Hypertension • Hypokalemia

Primary hyperaldosteronism (PHA), also known as *Conn's disease* or *primary aldosteronism*, was first described in humans in 1955[1] and in cats in 1983.[2] Since that time, sporadic case reports have appeared in the literature describing feline PHA, either as the sole pathology,[3–7] with other endocrinopathies,[8] or in association with neoplastic abnormalities.[9] In humans, PHA was an uncommon diagnosis but is now recognized as the most common cause of endocrine hypertension, the most frequent cause of secondary hypertension. Although debate exists over the best way to diagnose PHA in humans, recent studies suggest that 5% to 13% of patients who have hypertension experience PHA.[10–13] Similar to early underrecognition in human hypertension, because blood pressure is not always considered part of the minimum database for routine physical assessment of healthy or diseased cats, and because aldosterone is not routinely measured in all cases of feline hypertension, cats may also experience PHA more commonly than is reported.

ALDOSTERONE PHYSIOLOGY

The principal known function of aldosterone is regulation of systemic blood pressure and homeostasis of extracellular fluid volume in response to changes in hemodynamics and electrolytes. Aldosterone acts by increasing secretion of potassium and hydrogen and resorption of sodium and chloride in the distal nephrons of the kidneys. Thus, increased plasma aldosterone concentrations cause increases in sodium concentration and volume of the extracellular fluid.

Aldosterone production in the zona glomerulosa of the adrenal cortex is regulated by the renin–angiotensin system (also called the *renin–angiotensin–aldosterone system*; RAAS) and extracellular potassium concentrations.[14] The kidneys increase renin secretion in response to a decrease in circulating blood volume or renal blood flow sensed by the juxtaglomerular apparatus. Decreased delivery of sodium and chloride to the macula densa cells in the distal tubules also stimulates renin secretion. Renin cleaves angiotensinogen, produced by the liver, into angiotensin I, which is hydrolyzed to angiotensin II by angiotensin-converting enzyme (ACE). In addition to

Animal Specialty Group, 4641 Colorado Boulevard, Los Angeles, CA 90039, USA
E-mail address: rhondaschulman@gmail.com

Vet Clin Small Anim 40 (2010) 353–359
doi:10.1016/j.cvsm.2009.10.006
0195-5616/10/$ – see front matter © 2010 Elsevier Inc. All rights reserved.

vetsmall.theclinics.com

being a powerful vasoconstrictor, angiotensin II stimulates aldosterone secretion. Potassium controls aldosterone secretion through a direct effect on the adrenal zona glomerulosa.[15]

Therefore, when the kidneys experience decreased blood flow, renin, angiotensin II, and aldosterone are increased, resulting in increased sodium retention, increased extracellular fluid volume, and lower extracellular concentrations of potassium (through loss in the urine). Once homeostasis is restored, renin production is reduced and the aldosterone concentration declines. In PHA, excess aldosterone causes systemic hypertension. The increased urinary loss of potassium may result in profound hypokalemia. As potassium shifts extracellularly, hydrogen ions move intracellularly. Metabolic alkalosis may result from the increased urinary loss of hydrogen ions in addition to the intracellular shift.[14]

PRIMARY HYPERALDOSTERONISM
Clinical Presentation

Cats diagnosed with PHA are usually geriatric, although one case study includes a cat as young as 5 years.[5] There do not appear to be sex or breed predilections. Weakness is the most common presenting sign, followed by cervical ventriflexion. The weakness may be acute in onset or more insidious in nature.[2,3,5–7,9] Hind limb weakness, episodic forelimb stiffness, and dysphagia were also described.[3] The weakness displayed by cats with PHA is typical of hypokalemic polymyopathy.[16] Hypokalemia in cats with PHA can also result in lethargy and depression.

Clinical signs related to systemic hypertension may be seen at initial presentation. Of 33 cats described in the literature, 11 presented with blindness caused by retinal detachment and intraocular hemorrhage.[2–4] Other consequences of systemic hypertension include myocardial hypertrophy and renal damage. Additional presenting signs include polyuria–polydipsia[3,4] and enuresis[4] weight loss,[4,8] diarrhea[7] and polyphagia.[3] Some cats with PHA have palpable abdominal masses.[4,5]

Biochemical abnormalities found in cats with PHA are consistent with the excessive circulating concentrations of aldosterone. Moderate-to-severe degrees of hypokalemia are typically seen, whereas serum sodium concentrations may be normal or mildly increased.[2–9,17] It is not surprising that the serum sodium concentrations are only mildly increased, if at all, given the increased water resorption that accompanies the aldosterone-driven sodium resorption.[18] Early in the disease course, serum potassium concentrations may be normal.[19] Urinary fractional excretion of potassium is greatly increased because of the effects of aldosterone. Serum creatinine kinase concentrations are also usually markedly elevated, secondary to hypokalemic polymyopathy.[20]

Cats with PHA may have evidence of renal disease, including isosthenuria and increases in serum creatinine and BUN concentrations. Hyperaldosteronism may lead to hyaline arteriolar sclerosis, glomerular sclerosis, tubular atrophy, and interstitial fibrosis, thus causing or worsening chronic kidney disease.[19] Many hyperaldosteronemic cats that present without azotemia, or only mild azotemia, experience progression of renal disease.[2,3,19] In cases of adrenal tumors, plasma renin activity is typically low or absent because of negative feedback inhibition from excessive aldosterone. In some cases, renin escapes from suppression because excessive aldosterone results in continued activation of RAAS, progression of renal disease caused by hypertension, and additional damage from excess angiotensin II.[19,21] Humans with hyperaldosteronism often develop renal cysts and proteinuria. The proteinuria of hyperaldosteronism is of greater magnitude than that seen with primary hypertension.[12,21–23]

In human medicine, the adverse effects of aldosterone on the cardiovascular system are well established. Aldosterone excess leads to left ventricular hypertrophy and cardiac fibrosis. These changes are more severe than with primary hypertension. Humans who have aldosteronism are at increased risk for cardiac arrhythmias.[11,22] Many cats diagnosed with hyperaldosteronism had evidence of cardiovascular disease, including cardiac murmurs, radiographic cardiomegaly, or ventricular hypertrophy noted on echocardiogram[4–8]; the role of the hyperaldosteronism in the generation or progression of cardiac disease in cats is unknown.

Hyperaldosteronism is also implicated in metabolic syndrome, which is characterized by insulin resistance, impaired beta-cell function, excessive proinflammatory proteins, and a prothrombotic tendency.[22,24] Humans who have metabolic syndrome are at far greater risk for overt diabetes mellitus, heart disease, and stroke. Further work is needed to establish a similar metabolic syndrome in cats.

Etiology

In humans, six different subtypes of PHA have been identified. Patients most commonly experience either bilateral idiopathic hyperaldosteronism or an aldosterone-producing adenoma. Less commonly seen causes of PHA in humans include unilateral adrenal hyperplasia and familial hyperaldosteronism (FH), of which two forms, FH type I and FH type II, have been described.[25]

In cats with PHA, most cases are attributed to either adrenal adenomas or carcinomas. Of 23 cases reported in the literature with histopathologic examination of the affected adrenal glands, 11 developed hyperaldosteronism associated with unilateral carcinoma[2–4,7,8,17]; 9 were diagnosed with adenomas[3,5,9]; and 2 of 9 had bilateral disease.[3] Additionally, in one report 3 cats were diagnosed with bilateral adrenal hyperplasia.[19]

Feline PHA has also been diagnosed as part of other conditions. One cat had an adrenal carcinoma, which produced excessive amounts of both aldosterone and progesterone.[8] Another cat had PHA diagnosed as part of multiple endocrine neoplasia I (MEN I). MEN is a well-recognized group of autosomal dominant syndromes in which single human patients develop multiple tumors originating in endocrine organs. The MEN I syndrome usually involves the pancreas, parathyroid glands, and pituitary gland. Adrenocortical neoplasia is found in 13% to 40% of humans who have MEN I. The cat described by Reimer and colleagues[9] was diagnosed with an adrenal adenoma, pancreatic insulin-secreting tumor, and a parathyroid gland adenoma.

Diagnosis

When Conn[1] first described primary hyperaldosteronism in 1955, he discussed three hallmarks: hypertension, hypokalemia, and increased serum aldosterone concentration. In contrast, in secondary hyperaldosteronism, the increase in aldosterone concentration results from a primary increase in renin. Secondary hyperaldosteronism is most often associated with renal disease, cardiovascular disease, and liver failure.[26]

In veterinary patients, hyperaldosteronism is usually suspected in cats with hypokalemia and hypertension (often refractory) for which another cause cannot be identified. Hypokalemia can result from various disorders, including renal failure, hepatic dysfunction, infection, gastrointestinal disease, cardiac disease, and endocrinopathies such as hyperthyroidism and diabetes mellitus.[27] A thorough history, physical examination, and minimum database consisting of a complete blood cell count, chemistry profile, and urinalysis will rule out most causes of hypokalemia. Similarly, systemic hypertension can have various causes in the cat, with renal disease and hyperthyroidism among the most common.[28]

Traditionally, for Conn's disease in humans, hypokalemia was a necessary finding on screening tests before additional diagnostic testing. This prerequisite resulted in underrecognition of PHA in humans who had hypertension. Currently, hypokalemia is rarely seen in human PHA or found only late in the disease course.[10,13,25] Similarly, some cats with PHA do not display hypokalemia on initial presentation.

In the 2005 paper by Javadi and colleagues,[19] 5 of 11 cats with PHA had normal serum potassium concentrations, although 2 did develop hypokalemia. Hypokalemia may represent a much later development in the natural course of the disease. Failure to suspect PHA because of normal potassium results on screening tests may result in underdiagnosis of feline PHA in the hypertensive feline population, and delay in identification and management of individual patients.

Increased aldosterone concentration is the diagnostic hallmark of PHA, both in cats and humans. In humans, aldosterone is measured under controlled conditions. Variables that are controlled include amount of salt in the diet, administration of antihypertensive medications, and patient position at blood draw.[13] In a group of healthy cats, Javadi and colleagues[29] described a reference range for plasma aldosterone concentration of 80 to 450 pmol/L (28.8–162.2 pg/mL), which was consistent with human measurements from that same laboratory. Stress and body position did not affect aldosterone concentrations in cats.

Serum aldosterone measurement is widely available at veterinary laboratories. Veterinarians should observe reference ranges provided by the specific laboratory. Patient aldosterone concentrations are interpreted in combination with serum potassium concentrations. Because potassium is a major stimulus for aldosterone secretion, hypokalemia is a potent suppressor of aldosterone secretion in the normal animal. Among some cats with PHA in Javadi's study, aldosterone concentrations fell within the reference ranges; however, the investigators concluded that the aldosterone concentrations were inappropriately high in light of the concurrent hypokalemia.[19] Therefore, if an aldosterone concentration is in the high-normal range, but the potassium concentration is low, PHA should still be considered.

Recently, a reference range for the urinary aldosterone:creatinine ratio (UACR) was established for cats. The UACR offers advantages over plasma aldosterone concentrations in that it provides an indication of circulating aldosterone concentrations over time (the time over which the urine is made) without requiring frequent blood sampling or protracted urine collections.[30] The efficacy of the UACR in cats with spontaneously occurring PHA requires further examination.

In cats with hyperaldosteronemia and hypertension, plasma renin activity should be measured to differentiate primary from secondary hyperaldosteronism. In primary hyperaldosteronism, plasma renin activity is minimal, reflecting the autonomous secretion of aldosterone by the adrenal glands.[26] In humans, the aldosterone:renin ratio (ARR) is used as the primary screening test for PHA. In both humans and cats, cases of PHA have been reported with normal plasma renin activity, complicating definitive diagnosis.[19,21]

Hypothetically, in cats with less extremely high aldosterone, such as those with adrenal adenoma rather than adrenal neoplasia, plasma renin activity may remain normal. Cats with severe hyperaldosteronism should have more consistent and measurable suppression of plasma renin activity.[19] Aging and neutering may also decrease plasma renin activity in healthy cats, thus causing the ARR to be higher.[29] Unfortunately, measurements of renin activity are not widely available through veterinary laboratories and clinicians often must rely on aldosterone measurement as a solitary test. PHA is often confirmed retrospectively after surgical removal of an adrenal tumor and subsequent dramatic decline in aldosterone concentrations.[8]

Imaging of the adrenal glands is frequently performed in veterinary patients with PHA. Ultrasound findings in cats include adrenal mass, adrenal calcification, and changes in echogenicity.[3-9,17,19] CT and MRI have also been used to improve imaging of the adrenal glands in cats.[3,17,19] Of 25 cases with reported advanced imaging, only 2 had normal-appearing adrenal glands on ultrasound or CT.[19] However, the finding of an enlarged adrenal gland or adrenal mass does not mean that it is producing excessive aldosterone. Adrenal masses in the cat are often incidental findings known as *incidentalomas*; other adrenal masses in cats can be attributed to hypercortisolism (cortisol-secreting), pheochromocytomas, and progesterone-secreting tumors.[7,8] In contrast to cats, adrenal imaging is performed in human patients only after PHA is diagnosed; imaging is used to help differentiate between unilateral adenomas and bilateral hyperplasia. Most adenomas identified in humans are smaller than 10 to 20 mm and can escape detection with CT and MRI.[31]

Testing for primary aldosteronism in humans occurs in three phases: case-finding, confirmation, and subtype evaluation. Case-finding testing involves screening of the hypertensive population most likely to experience PHA (unexplained hypokalemia, resistant hypertension, early-onset hypertension, adrenal mass). Screening is typically performed using the ARR. If that test is positive, patients are then confirmed to have PHA using an exclusion test. Exclusion tests suppress aldosterone secretion and are used to rule out false-positives. These tests include those for oral sodium loading, saline infusion, fludrocortisone with salt loading, and captopril.[13,25,32]

Oral sodium loading was found to be not successful in cats (it did not increase the amount of sodium in the urine in more than half of the cats), nor did oral sodium loading decrease aldosterone secretion. Fludrocortisone administration suppressed urinary aldosterone secretion in three normal cats but not in one cat with confirmed PHA, and therefore may be a useful tool.[30] Other aldosterone-suppression testing has not been examined for validity in cats. Subtype evaluation is performed in humans to distinguish between idiopathic bilateral adrenal hyperplasia, which is treated medically, and unilateral adenomas, which are treated surgically, and to differentiate the more uncommon subtypes of PHA. Adrenal vein sampling is considered the gold standard for documenting lateralization of aldosterone secretion, and thus deciding whether surgery should be considered.[31]

Treatment and Prognosis

For cats with unilateral disease, surgical removal of the affected adrenal gland remains preferred treatment. Surgery seems to be curative for both adenomas and carcinomas, with signs of hypokalemia and hypertension resolving without further treatment.[3-5,7] Cats surviving the immediate postoperative period often had survival times of many years.[3] Cats with carcinomas seem to have a similarly good postsurgical prognosis, as do those with adenomas.[3] Invasion of the caudal vena cava from an adrenal tumor, or associated thrombosis is usually considered a contraindication to surgery, but successful outcomes have been reported even with vena cava thrombosis.[7] In humans who have unilateral adenomas, surgery is the recommended treatment. Removing the affected adrenal gland has been shown to normalize the RAAS and cure hypokalemia.[22,31] Additionally, systemic hypertension is improved in all patients and cured in up to 82%.[31]

Cats may also do well with medical management, which consists of spironolactone therapy, potassium supplementation, and antihypertensive drugs as needed. Spironolactone is an aldosterone antagonist that binds to the aldosterone receptors in the distal convoluted tubules. Reported survival times for cats treated medically often range from many months to years.[3,4] A newer-generation aldosterone antagonist, eplerenone, is being examined for use in humans who have PHA. In humans, side effects may arise from spironolactone's affinity for androgen, estrogen, and progesterone receptors. Eplerenone has a far diminished affinity for these other receptors.[11] Whether this drug would be suitable for use in cats is unknown.

SUMMARY

PHA is being recognized more frequently in cats. Usual hallmarks of the disease include hypokalemia and systemic hypertension. Ultrasound frequently detects an abnormality in the affected adrenal gland. Diagnosis is based on increased plasma or serum aldosterone concentrations, particularly in the face of hypokalemia and low renin activity (when measurement is available). Cats with PHA have good prognoses with surgical excision of tumor-bearing adrenal glands. Medical management can stabilize patients for many months. The reported incidence is unlikely to increase as practitioners become more aware of the condition and diagnose it earlier in the disease course. If veterinarians choose to use humans as an experimental model, PHA should be considered a differential for cats with hypertension of unknown cause or that is refractory to treatment. Using hypokalemia as a definitive criterion in screening for PHA may result in late-stage diagnosis and underrecognition of incidence of PHA in the hypertensive population, and may also explain the discrepancy in the size of the adrenal glands in affected humans (often <10–20 mm) and cats (enlarged enough to be detected by ultrasonography). Adrenal carcinoma seems to be a far more frequent cause of PHA in cats than in humans, but carries a far better prognosis in cats.

REFERENCES

1. Conn JW. Presidential address: part 1: painting background. Part II: primary aldosteronism, a new clinical syndrome. J Lab Clin Med 1955;45:3–17.
2. Eger CE, Robinson WF, Huxtable CR. Primary aldosteronism (Conn's syndrome) in a cat; a case report and review of comparative aspects. J Small Anim Pract 1983;24:293–307.
3. Ash RA, Harvey AM, Tasker S. Primary hyperaldosteronism in the cat; a series of 13 cases. J Feline Med Surg 2005;7:173–82.
4. Flood SM, Randolph JF, Gelzer AR, et al. Primary hyperaldosteronism in two cats. J Am Anim Hosp Assoc 1999;35:411–6.
5. MacKay AD, Holt PE, Sparkes AH. Successful surgical treatment of a cat with primary hyperaldosteronism. J Feline Med Surg 1999;1:117–22.
6. Moore LE, Biller DS, Smith TA. Use of abdominal ultrasonography in the diagnosis of primary hyperaldosteronism in a cat. J Am Vet Med Assoc 2000;217:213–5.
7. Rose SA, Kyles AE, Labelle P, et al. Adrenalectomy and caval thrombectomy in a cat with primary hyperaldosteronism. J Am Anim Hosp Assoc 2007;43:209–14.
8. DeClue AE, Breshears LA, Pardo ID, et al. Hyperaldosteronism and hyperprogesteronism in a cat with an adrenal cortical carcinoma. J Vet Intern Med 2005;19: 355–8.
9. Reimer SB, Pelosi A, Frank JD, et al. Multiple endocrine neoplasia type I in a cat. J Am Vet Med Assoc 2005;227:101–4.
10. Calhoun DA. Is there an unrecognized epidemic of primary aldosteronism? (pro). Hypertension 2007;50:447–53.
11. Karagiannis A, Tziomalos K, Kakafika AI, et al. Medical treatment as an alternative to adrenalectomy in patients with aldosterone-producing adenomas. Endocr Relat Cancer 2008;15:693–700.

12. Rossi GP, Bernini G, Desideri G, et al. Renal damage in primary aldosteronism: results of the PAPY study. Hypertension 2006;48:232–8.

13. Rossi GP, Seccia TM, Pessina AC. Primary aldosteronism- part I: prevalence, screening, and selection of cases for adrenal vein sampling. J Nephrol 2008; 21:447–54.

14. Feldman EC, Nelson RW. Renal hormones and atrial natriuretic hormone. In: Canine and feline endocrinology and reproduction. 3rd edition. Pennsylvania: Saunders; 2003. p. 746–9.

15. Reusch CE. Hyperadrenocorticism in cats. In: Ettinger SJ, Feldman EC, editors. Textbook of veterinary internal medicine. 6th edition. Pennsylvania: Elsevier Saunders; 2004. p. 1610–3.

16. Dow SW, LeCouteyr RA, Fettman MJ, et al. Potassium depletion in cats: hypokalemic polymyopathy. J Am Vet Med Assoc 1987;191:1563–8.

17. Rijnberk A, Voorhout G, Kooistra HS, et al. Hyperaldosteronism in a cat with metastasized adrenocortical tumour. Vet Q 2001;23:38–43.

18. Guyton AC. Adrenocortical hormones. In: Textbook of medical physiology. Pennsylvania: WB Saunders Company; 2006. p. 944–50.

19. Javadi S, Djajadiningrat-Laanen SC, Kooistra HS, et al. Primary hyperaldosteronism, a mediator of progressive renal disease in cats. Domest Anim Endocrinol 2005;28:85–104.

20. Ahn A. Hyperaldosteronism in cats. Semin Vet Med Surg 1994;9:153–7.

21. Catena C, Colussi G, Chiuch A, et al. Relationships of plasma renin levels with renal function in patients with primary aldosteronism. Clin J Am Soc Nephrol 2007;2(4):722–31.

22. Giacchetti G, Turchi F, Boscaro M, et al. Management of primary aldosteronism: its complications and their outcomes after treatment. Curr Vasc Pharmacol 2009; 7(2):244–9.

23. Sechi LA, Novello M, Lapenna R, et al. Long-term renal outcomes in patients with primary aldosteronism. JAMA 2006;295:2638–45.

24. Sowers JR, Whaley-Connell A, Epstein M. Narrative review: the emerging clinical implications of the role of aldosterone in the metabolic syndrome and resistant hypertension. Ann Intern Med 2009;150:776–83.

25. Young WF. Minireview: primary aldosteronism-changing concepts in diagnosis and treatment. Endocrinology 2003;144:2208–13.

26. Conn JW, Cohen EL, Rovner DR. Suppression of plasma renin activity in primary aldosteronism. JAMA 1964;190:213–21.

27. Dow SW, Fettman MJ, Curtis CR, et al. Hypokalemia in cats: 186 cases (1984–1987). J Am Vet Med Assoc 1989;194:1604–8.

28. Brown SA. Pathophysiology of systemic hypertension. In: Ettinger SJ, Feldman EC, editors. Textbook of veterinary internal medicine. 6th edition. Pennsylvania: Elsevier Saunders; 2004. p. 472–3.

29. Javadi S, Slingerland LI, van de Beek MG, et al. Plasma renin activity and plasma concentrations of aldosterone, cortisol, adrenocorticotropic hormone and alpha-melanocyte-stimulating hormone in healthy cats. J Vet Intern Med 2004;18:625–31.

30. Djajadiningrat-Laanen SC, Galac S, Cammelbeeck SE, et al. Urinary aldosterone to creatinine ratio in cats before and after suppression with salt or fludrocortisone acetate. J Vet Intern Med 2008;22:1283–8.

31. Rossi GP, Seccia TM, Pessina AC. Primary aldosteronism- part II: subtype differentiation and treatment. J Nephrol 2008;21:455–62.

32. Young WF. Primary aldosteronism: renaissance of a syndrome. Clin Endocrinol 2007;66:607–18.

Index

Note: Page numbers of article titles are in **boldface** type.

Vet Clin Small Anim 40 (2010) 361–368
doi:10.1016/S0195-5616(10)00012-4
0195-5616/10/$ – see front matter © 2010 Elsevier Inc. All rights reserved.

vetsmall.theclinics.com

Moving?

Make sure your subscription moves with you!

To notify us of your new address, find your **Clinics Account Number** (located on your mailing label above your name), and contact customer service at:

Email: journalscustomerservice-usa@elsevier.com

800-654-2452 (subscribers in the U.S. & Canada)
314-447-8871 (subscribers outside of the U.S. & Canada)

Fax number: 314-447-8029

Elsevier Health Sciences Division
Subscription Customer Service
3251 Riverport Lane
Maryland Heights, MO 63043

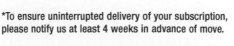

Moving?

Make sure your subscription moves with you!

To notify us of your new address, find your Clinics Account Number (located on your mailing label above your name), and contact customer service at:

Email: journalscustomerservice-usa@elsevier.com

800-654-2452 (subscribers in the U.S. & Canada)
314-447-8871 (subscribers outside of the U.S. & Canada)

Fax number: 314-447-8029

Elsevier Health Sciences Division
Subscription Customer Service
3251 Riverport Lane
Maryland Heights, MO 63043

To ensure uninterrupted delivery of your subscription, please notify us at least 4 weeks in advance of move.

Printed and bound by CPI Group (UK) Ltd, Croydon, CR0 4YY

03/10/2024

01040459-0014